£3.

Paediatric and Neonatal Anaesthesia

Anaesthesia in a Nutshell

Commissioning Editor: Michael Parkinson
Project Development Manager: Clive Hewat
Project Manager: Frances Affleck
Designer: George Ajayi

Paediatric and Neonatal Anaesthesia

Anaesthesia in a Nutshell

Dr Ann E Black MB BS FRCA
Consultant Paediatric Anaesthetist
Great Ormond Street Hospital for Children
London, UK

Dr Angus McEwan MB CHB FRCA
Consultant Paediatric Anaesthetist
Great Ormond Street Hospital for Children
London, UK

Series Editors: Neville Robinson and George Hall

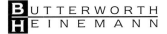
BUTTERWORTH
HEINEMANN

Edinburgh London New York Oxford Philadelphia St Louis Sydney Toronto 2004

BUTTERWORTH-HEINEMANN
An imprint of Elsevier Limited
© 2004, Elsevier Limited. All rights reserved.

First published 2004

ISBN 0750653809

British Library Cataloguing in Publication Data
A catalogue record for this book is available from the British Library

Library of Congress Cataloging in Publication Data
A catalog record for this book is available from the Library of Congress

Notice
Medical knowledge is constantly changing. Standard safety precautions must be followed, but as new research and clinical experience broaden our knowledge, changes in treatment and drug therapy may become necessary or appropriate. Readers are advised to check the most current product information provided by the manufacturer of each drug to be administered to verify the recommended dose, the method and duration of administration, and contraindications. It is the responsibility of the practitioner, relying on experience and knowledge of the patient, to determine dosages and the best treatment for each individual patient. Neither the Publisher nor the authors assumes any liability for any injury and/or damage to persons or property arising from this publication.

The Publisher

 your source for books,
journals and multimedia
in the health sciences

www.elsevierhealth.com

The
Publisher's
policy is to use
**paper manufactured
from sustainable forests**

Printed in China

Contents

Series preface

Specialist registrars and senior house officers in anaesthesia are now trained by the use of modular educational programmes. In these short periods of intense training, the anaesthetist must acquire a fundamental understanding of each anaesthetic speciality. To meet these needs, the trainee requires a concise, pocket-sized book that contains the core knowledge of each subject.

The aims of these 'nutshell' guides are two-fold: first, to provide trainees with the fundamental information necessary for the understanding and safe practice of anaesthesia in each speciality; and, second, to cover all the key areas of the fellowship examination of the Royal College of Anaesthetists and so act as revision guides for trainees.

P. N. Robinson
G. M. Hall

Preface

Our aim in writing this book has been to provide both the background information required for studying paediatric anaesthesia, and sufficient practical information for those anaesthetists seeking to provide anaesthesia for children.

Modern modular training programmes compress sub-specialty training limiting the exposure to different anaesthetic experiences. The training programmes also demand the gathering of skills and information within a short period of time. Rather than replicate larger and very informative paediatric textbooks, we have deliberately concentrated on covering core knowledge, with chapters reflecting all sub-specialist areas which we hope will allow a ready reference for most paediatric cases required for anaesthetists both during training and in practice. The book seeks to provide trainees with a clear understanding of the important issues regarding the care of children – from their preoperative preparation and consent to their wider perioperative care.

There has been rapid development in delivery of anaesthetic care outside the anaesthetic room and this challenging area has also been addressed. In addition we have added a section on common medical conditions which are relevant to paediatric anaesthetists. To reflect the huge amount of useful information that is now available on the World Wide Web we have included useful paediatric sites.

We have found our work with children and their families challenging but hugely rewarding and we hope that this book will help readers gain confidence and skills rapidly so that they too can enjoy the practice of paediatric anaesthesia.

We would like to thank the editorial team, particularly Clive Hewat and Professor George Hall who have been patient and understanding throughout the project.

1

Physiology and anatomy relevant to paediatric anaesthesia

The cardiovascular system
Foetal and neonatal and circulation

Gas exchange in the fetus takes place via the low-resistance placental circulation, which receives 40% of the foetal cardiac output.

Blood from the right ventricle is directed away from the pulmonary circulation through the patent foramen ovale (PFO) and patent ductus arteriosus (PDA). Only a small proportion of the cardiac output (5–10%) goes to the high-resistance circulation of the foetal lungs. Most blood goes to the placental circulation where it is oxygenated and carbon dioxide is removed. About one-third of the oxygenated blood returning from the placenta via the ductus venosus and inferior vena cava (IVC) is directed through the PFO to the left atrium (Fig 1.1). This blood is combined with the small amount of blood returning from the lungs and is then directed by the left ventricle up the ascending aorta to the cerebral, coronary and upper limb circulation. Less well-oxygenated blood from the superior vena cava (SVC), the liver and gut passes to the right atrium, right ventricle and pulmonary artery. Due to the high pulmonary vascular resistance, it is directed down the PDA to the descending aorta, so supplying the abdominal organs, lower limbs and placenta. The foetal right ventricle is responsible for about two-thirds of the cardiac output while the left ventricle contributes one-third.

Changes at birth

In the foetus, the lungs are fluid filled and only 40% expanded. At birth, the lungs quickly expand and fill with air as a result of negative intrapleural pressures. Blood flow to the placenta decreases rapidly, the umbilical cord is clamped and blood flow ceases. At the same time, pulmonary blood flow increases as the pulmonary vascular resistance decreases due to:

- an increase in alveolar PO_2
- a decrease in alveolar PCO_2

- physical expansion of the lungs widening the calibre of the blood vessels.

As blood flow to the lungs increases other changes occur (Fig 1.2):

- Blood flow from the lungs to the pulmonary veins and left atrium increases, resulting in an increase in left arterial pressure which causes the flap-like foramen ovale to close.
- Right atrial pressure decreases as umbilical flow ceases when flow from the placenta to the IVC stops.
- Systemic vascular resistance increases as the low-resistance placental circulation is lost.
- Aortic pressure increases and flow in the ductus arteriosus is reversed and becomes left to right.
- As the ductus arteriosus is perfused with oxygenated blood, it begins to constrict. Although the exact mechanism is not fully understood, it is mediated by prostaglandins. It may take several days for the duct to close completely.

Transitional circulation
During foetal life, the pulmonary arteries are exposed to systemic pressures through the PDA and have muscular walls. In the early neonatal period, the pulmonary arteries remain very sensitive to the vasoconstrictor effects of hypoxaemia, acidosis and serotonin, and to the vasodilator effects of acetylcholine and nitric oxide.

Under certain conditions, the ductus arteriosus may reopen creating a **transitional circulation** with right-to-left shunting, which results in increased hypoxaemia. This situation is associated with the following conditions:

- congenital diaphragmatic hernia
- respiratory distress syndrome
- cardiac failure
- surgical stress
- sepsis
- hypoxaemia
- acidosis.

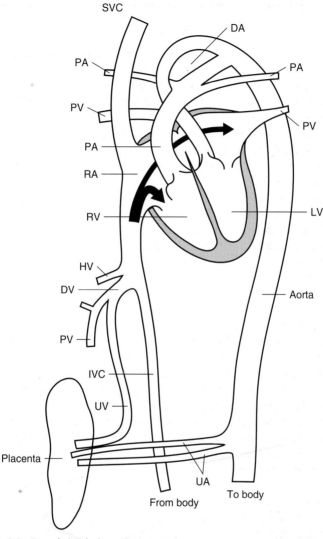

Figure 1.1 Foetal circulation – SVC, superior vena cava; PA, pulmonary artery; PV, pulmonary vein; DA, ductus arteriosus; RA, right atrium; LV, left ventricle; RV, right ventricle; HV, hepatic vein; DV, ductus venosus; PV, portal vein; IVC, inferior vena cava; UV, umbilical vein; UA, umbilical artery. (After Comroe JH. Physiology of respiration, 2nd edn. Chicago: Year Book Medical Publishers; 1974, with permission.)

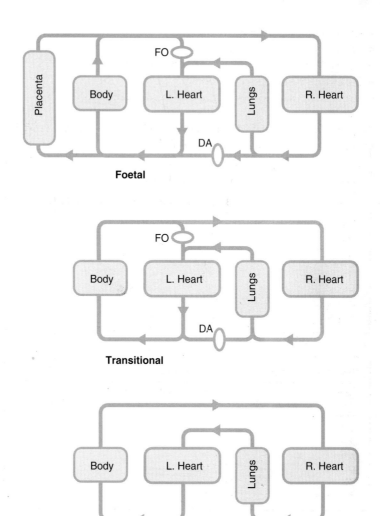

Figure 1.2 Physiological changes at birth – FO, foramen ovale; DA, ductus arteriosus. (After Hatch DJ, Sumner E. Textbook of paediatric anaesthetic practice. London: Bailliere Tindall; 1989, with permission.)

Myocardial function

Key differences between the neonatal myocardium and that of the adult are:

- ↓ contractile tissue (30% vs 60% in adult)
- less compliant

- relatively fixed stroke volume
- cardiac output is rate dependent
- relatively high myocardial oxygen consumption
- little myocardial functional reserve
- sensitive to calcium blocking agents (e.g. volatile agents)

The electrocardiogram shows marked right-axis deviation ($+180°$), which reduces to the adult value of $+90°$ by 6 months.

Box 1.1   Normal blood pressures in children

Age	Blood pressure (mmHg) systolic/diastolic
Preterm	49/24
Term	60/35
< 1 month	70/35
< 6 months	95/40
4 yr	95/55
6–8 yr	110/60
8–12 yr	115/65
12–16 yr	120/65

Box 1.2   Normal heart rates in children

Age	Heart rate (bpm)
Neonatal	100–170
< 1 yr	80–160
2 yr	80–130
4 yr	80–120
6–10 yr	75–115
10–14 yr	60–105
14–16 yr	55–100

At birth, the cardiac output is 300–400 ml/kg/min, which is equally distributed between the right and left ventricles. Therefore, the output of the left ventricle is doubled leaving little functional reserve. By 4 months, cardiac output has decreased to 200 ml/kg/min and the myocardium has greater functional reserve.

The neonatal myocardium cannot generate the same force as the adult myocardium and is less compliant (see Box 1.1). This is partly because the neonatal myocardium has less contractile tissue than the adult myocardium. In addition, the myofibrils and sarcoplasmic reticulum within the contractile tissue are immature. Calcium flux in the neonatal myocyte is less efficient than in the adult myocardium. This is thought to explain the sensitivity of the neonatal myocardium to calcium-blocking agents including halothane and isoflurane. The result is that the stroke volume is relatively fixed and the cardiac output is rate dependent (see Box 1.2). Bradycardia results in a dramatic fall in cardiac output and slow heart rates are poorly tolerated.

As neonates have a high oxygen consumption, hypoxaemia can develop rapidly. The neonatal response to hypoxia includes:

- bradycardia
- ↑ periperheral vascular resistance (PVR)
- ↑ systemic vascular resistance (SVR)
- risk of transitional circulation (see above).

Blood volume and oxygen transport

Neonatal blood volume is approximately 80 ml/kg but is higher in preterm babies, as shown in Box 1.3 (90–95 ml/kg). However, this may vary by as much as 20% in the early postnatal period, depending on the amount of maternal/foetal transfusion. Neonates may be hypovolaemic if foetal hypoxia has been severe resulting in vasoconstriction and a smaller blood volume.

Box 1.3   Blood volumes in children

Age	Blood volume (ml/kg)
Preterm	90–95
Term	80–85
< 2 yr	75
> 2 yr	70

Systolic blood pressure is a reliable reflection of intravascular blood volume. Neonates have little ability to compensate for blood loss, probably due to the combination of immature baroreceptor responses, poor capacitance of blood vessels, and a limited reserve in cardiac output.

The haemoglobin concentration of 17 g/dl at birth decreases to 11 g/dl over the next 4–8 weeks, and the fall is greater in preterm babies. This physiological anaemia is due to reduced red cell production because of better tissue oxygenation after birth and also because of a reduction in red cell survival. Most haemoglobin at birth is foetal (HbF). This has a higher affinity for oxygen than adult haemoglobin (HbA), and releases oxygen less readily. The p50 of HbF is 2.7 kPa compared with 3.6 kPa for HbA. This high affinity is compensated for by the relatively greater acidosis, hypercapnia and hypoxia in the peripheral tissues, which shifts the oxygen dissociation curve to the right. By 3 months, the HbF has largely been replaced by HbA.

The respiratory system
Anatomy
Key features of neonatal airway anatomy are:

- The neonate or young infant has a relatively large head, protruding occiput and short neck.
- The tongue is large and the larynx lies more anterior and cephalad at the level of C4 rather than C6 as in adults. During larygoscopy, the conventional 'sniffing the morning air position', which is used to help visualize the larynx in adult patients, is not helpful in babies because as the head is moved anteriorly so the larynx also moves anteriorly.
- The epiglottis is large, floppy and U-shaped, and a laryngoscope with a straight blade is often used to directly lift the epiglottis.
- The narrowest portion of the airway is at the level of the cricoid ring where local trauma from a tracheal tube may cause damage, particularly if the tube is too tight.
- The trachea is covered in ciliated pseudostratified epithelium which is loosely attached to underlying structures. Even relatively minor trauma to this epithelium can result in oedema formation under the epithelium which narrows the airway post-extubation therefore stridor is more common in neonates than older patients. As resistance to airflow in a tube increases with the fourth power of the radius of the tube, a small amount of oedema results in a large increase in resistance. In addition, long-term subglottic stenosis may occur as a result of damage to the area near the cricoid.
- The trachea is short, about 4–5 cm in length. It is very easy for the tracheal tube to be advanced into one or other of the main bronchi. If the tracheal tube is too short, it may be easily displaced from the larynx.
- The tracheal cartilages are soft and collapse easily with negative pressure during inspiration. The application of continuous positive airways pressure (CPAP) during spontaneous ventilation prevents their collapse, and also collapse of tissues in the pharynx and nasopharynx. CPAP is an important component of paediatric airway management.
- Neonates are frequently described as 'obligate nasal breathers'. This is probably not strictly true but they convert to mouth breathing only

slowly if the nasal passages are obstructed. Unfortunately, the nasal passages of neonates and infants are narrow and easily become blocked with secretions, swelling or even a nasogastric tube.

Physiology

Box 1.4   Key features of neonatal respiratory physiology

↑ Metabolic rate and oxygen consumption

Horizontal ribs (loss of bucket handle effect)

Breathing mainly diaphragmatic

Respiratory muscles prone to fatigue

Compliant chest wall

Relatively stiff lungs

↓ FRC

Closing volumes encroach on FRC

Alveolar ventilation :
  150 ml kg/min vs 60 ml/kg/min in adults

Alveolar ventilation: FRC 5 : 1 vs 1.5 : 1 in adults

↑ Respiratory rate

↓ Functional reserve

↑ Work of breathing

Development of the respiratory system

By 24 weeks gestation, respiratory bronchioles have formed, which allows gas exchange so the foetus is now viable. About the same time surfactant production begins.

Surfactant's role is to reduce surface tension, which permits alveoli to expand more easily and prevents their collapse. Pulmonary surfactants are phospholipids produced by type II pneumocytes; the main component is lecithin.

The maturity of foetal lungs can be gauged by measuring the lecithin/sphingomyelin ratio in amniotic fluid. The ratio increases with lung maturity from 1 at 32 weeks' gestation, 2 at 35 weeks' gestation, to 4–6 at term. Low surfactant levels can lead to respiratory distress syndrome which is characterized by atelectasis, ventilation/perfusion mismatch, stiff lungs with increased work of breathing and poor gas exchange. Various insults in the neonatal period can lead to reduced production of surfactant and these include hypoxia, hypothermia, acidosis and hyperoxia. In addition to surfactant production, the foetal lung produces a pulmonary fluid which fills the lungs and is thought to play a role in the normal development of the lung. During normal delivery, compression of the chest wall as the baby passes along the birth canal causes most of the fluid to be squeezed from the lungs. Any remaining fluid must be removed by the lymphatic drainage. Babies born by Caesarean section do not have the same high intrathoracic pressure applied and consequently have a greater amount of fluid in the lungs after birth. The neonatal lung has relatively few alveoli at birth and gas exchange occurs via transitory ducts and saccules. However, alveoli proliferation occurs after birth and continues into childhood.

Control of breathing
Foetal breathing starts early in gestation and is important for the normal development of the lungs and respiratory muscles.

- Breathing in the neonate is controlled by the integration of impulses from central and peripheral chemoreceptors and by mechanical receptors in the lung and chest wall. Control of breathing is well developed in full-term neonates but is different from adults.
- The high metabolic rate and oxygen consumption of neonates is reflected in increased ventilation requirements.
- The increase in breathing in response to hypercapnia is less in neonates than in older infants and is less sustained. Both prematurity and hypoxaemia reduce this response further.

Research has shown that administering hypoxic gas mixtures to neonates produces an initial increase in ventilation, but a subsequent respiratory depression. This biphasic response to hypoxia is not seen in older children or adults who respond to hypoxia with an increase in ventilation. Peripheral chemoreceptors are responsible for the initial increase in ventilation, while a central mechanism is implicated in the later respiratory depression.

Hypothermia abolishes this biphasic response and respiratory depression is the first response seen. Hypoxic neonates are more prone to apnoea and the administration of oxygen is protective.

The intermittent breathing of the foetus may continue into the neonatal period and is known as periodic breathing. It is characterized by short periods of apnoea lasting up to 10 sec which are not associated with cyanosis or bradycardia. This periodic breathing is normal and poses no threat. However, more sinister are apnoeas that last for longer than 20 sec, or are associated with cyanosis or bradycardia. The origin of these apnoeas may be central or obstructive, and can result from other conditions such as sepsis, hypothermia or simply be associated with prematurity. Neonates are more prone to apnoea after general anaesthesia and those under 46 weeks' postgestational age are thought to be at greatest risk.

Lung mechanics
The following are key differences in neonates:

- The ribs are almost horizontal and the 'bucket handle' action of the ribs in adults, which increases the anterior to posterior distance, does not occur in neonates.
- Breathing is predominately diaphragmatic; any increase in intra-abdominal pressure can reduce the diaphragmatic excursion and thus tidal breathing.
- The preterm or neonatal diaphragm is prone to fatigue because it contains only a small proportion of the type 1 muscle fibres: 10% in the preterm diaphragm rising to 30% in the full-term infant and to the adult level of 50–60% by 1 year of age.
- The chest wall is very compliant in the new born and total compliance of the chest approximates to lung compliance. The chest wall is easily deformed during contraction of the diaphragm resulting in a paradoxical breathing pattern. Paradoxical breathing is particularly marked during REM sleep and during anaesthesia when the intercostal muscles, which usually act to reinforce the chest wall, are relaxed or when any obstruction to ventilation occurs.
- The lungs are stiff at birth partly because of residual fluid, but compliance slowly increases.
- The functional residual capacity (FRC) of the lung is low in the neonate because of the combination of the compliant chest wall and the elastic recoil of the lungs which allows the lungs to rest at small volumes. In addition, the closing volume is large, allowing the closing volume to encroach on FRC even during normal tidal breathing. This can lead to small airway closure with intrapulmonary shunting and a decrease in arterial oxygen tension. This is more common during and after anaesthesia because of a decrease in FRC. These effects are most marked in small, preterm infants and in those with hyaline membrane disease.
- FRC is maintained in the neonate by a combination of high respiratory rate, early termination of expiration, laryngeal narrowing to produce intrinsic CPAP and by the tone of the respiratory muscles. During anaesthesia, lung volumes are better maintained by using positive pressure ventilation, high respiratory rates, and positive end expiratory pressure or continuous positive airways pressure during spontaneous breathing.
- The total lung capacity (TLC) in a normal neonate is about 160 ml with the FRC accounting for about half this volume. The tidal volume is

approximately 16 ml and the dead space about 5 ml. These static lung volumes are in proportion to those in older children and in adults. The small absolute values have implications for anaesthetic breathing circuits and equipment which need to have small internal gas volumes. Alveolar ventilation, on the other hand, is much larger in neonates than in older children and adults, reflecting in part the higher metabolic rate and the increased oxygen consumption.

- In neonates, alveolar ventilation is about 150 ml/kg/min compared with 60 ml/kg/min in adults. Also, the ratio of alveolar ventilation to FRC is high (5 : 1) in neonates, compared with 1.5 : 1 in adults. Thus, the neonate has a reduced ventilatory reserve with a more rapid onset of hypoxaemia during anaesthesia if there is any respiratory obstruction.

- The work of breathing is the amount of energy expended to overcome the resistance in the airways and the elastic recoil of the lungs and chest wall. The most efficient respiratory rate in neonates is about 37 breaths/min and this uses 1% of the total energy expenditure.

Pain perception

The central nervous system of the neonate is different from that of the older child or adult. Myelination is incomplete, the nervous system is still developing, and reflexes and muscle tone are different. Examples of primitive reflexes include the rooting reflex, Moro reflex and grasp reflex. Until relatively recently, the immaturity of the CNS was thought to mean also that neonates did not feel pain in the same way as older children. This has now been shown to be incorrect and neonates may have an increased sensitivity to pain. Pain inflicted in the neonatal period may increase sensitivity to pain in later life. Neonates, including premature neonates, respond to painful stimuli with tachycardia, hypertension, a raised intracranial pressure and a neuroendocrine response. They also respond with crying, grimacing, increased muscle tone and drawing up of the legs. Some of these signs have been used to develop pain assessment tools for neonates and infants.

Aspects of intracranial physiology are dealt with in 'Anaesthesia for paediatric neurosurgery' (Chapter 12).

Renal function and fluid balance

Renal tubular function starts at around 9 weeks' gestation. During gestation, the developing kidneys produce dilute urine which contributes to the formation of the amniotic fluid. In the full-term neonate, formation of new nephrons is all but complete but, in the preterm infant, it continues into the neonatal period.

Neonatal renal function is characterized by:

- ↓ renal blood flow
- ↓ glomerular filtration rate (GFR)
- ↑ renal vascular resistance.

The high renal vascular resistance decreases in the first few weeks of life and this is reflected in the increased proportion of cardiac output perfusing the kidney, from 6% of cardiac output at birth to about 20% by 1 month.

The low GFR and reduced tubular function mean that the neonate handles water poorly and may easily become water overloaded. Also, the composition of urine remains relatively constant. Therefore, to excrete a solute load, the neonate requires sufficient water and this is even more important in preterm infants because of an increase in insensible water losses. The neonate is liable to hyponatraemia because sodium losses can be high and this is particularly likely if the infant has a high urine output. Glycosuria is more common in preterm infants because glucose reabsorption is limited.

Although plasma bicarbonate values are lower in neonates, the mechanism is unclear because the full-term neonate is able to effectively excrete acid. This ability is less well developed in the preterm neonate.

Total body water is greater in neonates and infants than in older children and adults, and the proportion of intra- to extracellular water also differs (see Box 1.5). The proportion of extracellular fluid decreases with age while the proportion of intracellular fluid increases with age.

Box 1.5 Intracellular to extracellular fluid at different ages (% of total body weight)

Fluid	Preterm	Term	Infant	Adult
ECF	50	40	30	20
ICF	30	35	35	45

Glucose metabolism

Immediate energy requirements in the first hours of life are provided by glycogen stores in the liver and heart. These stores are inadequate in both preterm infants and small for dates babies who are at risk of hypoglycaemia.

Hypoglycaemia can cause neurological damage and should be prevented by frequent measurement of blood glucose and by infusion of glucose 10%, if necessary.

Signs of hypoglycaemia in neonates include
- jitters
- convulsions
- apnoea.

Risk factors for hypoglycaemia in neonates
- sepsis
- hypothermia
- hypoxia
- prematurity
- small for gestational age
- infants of diabetic mothers.

Bilirubin metabolism

Physiological jaundice is relatively common in the term neonate due to the immaturity of the liver enzyme systems. Most bilirubin is unconjugated and is the result of:

- increased bilirubin production
- reduced hepatic uptake
- reduced intrahepatic conjugation.

Jaundice usually resolves in the first few days or weeks without any problem. Concentrations of bilirubin are usually relatively low (< 100 µmol/l) and do not cause any neurological damage because the blood–brain barrier in the term infant is protective. However, brain damage can occur with high levels of bilirubin or at lower levels if the protective blood–brain barrier is disrupted.

The blood–brain barrier is less effective in the presence of:

- prematurity
- sepsis
- hypothermia
- hypoxia
- acidosis
- hypoalbuminaemia (less protein binding).

Treatment of jaundice includes phototherapy and sometimes exchange transfusion.

Temperature regulation

Neonates, particularly preterm neonates and those small for dates, are prone to hypothermia if placed in a cool environment. This is primarily because they have a large surface area to body weight ratio and lack subcutaneous fat.

Mechanisms of heat loss include
- radiation
- conduction
- convection
- evaporation.

Neonates do not have the ability to shiver and heat production in neonates is by 'non-shivering thermogenesis'. The energy is derived from the metabolism of brown fat located around the scapulae, kidneys and mediastinum. Brown fat accounts for up to 6% of the neonate's total body weight. It has a rich blood and sympathetic supply and its metabolism is stimulated by release of noradrenaline from these nerve endings. Heat production results in an increase in oxygen and glucose consumption with lactate production, all of which are detrimental in sick infants with marginal physiological reserves. Peripheral vasoconstriction occurs in response to cooling and this results in a core to periphery temperature gradient. To prevent metabolic responses to cold, a sick infant should be nursed in a neutral thermal environment. This is an ambient temperature in which no metabolic response from the baby is required to stay warm. This varies from 35°C for very small babies in the first hours of life, to 29°C in 4-week-old babies.

During anaesthesia, the normal regulatory responses of peripheral vasoconstriction and increased heat production are abolished and infants cool very quickly as heat is redistributed to the periphery and then lost to the environment.

2

Pharmacology

Neonates, infants and young children handle drugs differently from older patients. The differences are most evident in neonates and the maturation of the processes involved is variable and unpredictable. Dose regimens need to be adjusted in amount and timing in the young and side effects may be greater.

Some drugs are relatively contraindicated:

- Propofol infusions (cardiac failure, increased sepsis and increased mortality).
- Aspirin (Reye's syndrome).
- Tetracycline (affects dentition).
- Verapamil (severe cardiac depression).
- Chloramphenicol (grey baby syndrome).

The management of premature infants is particularly challenging. They often require many drugs but have less metabolic activity and so are more likely to suffer side effects and adverse drug reactions.

Drugs can be given by many routes, and this flexibility is used more frequently in paediatric than adult practice. Common administration routes include oral, rectal, intramuscular, intravenous and inhalational. In addition, the buccal, nasal, transtracheal, subcutaneous and transcutaneous routes are used for some drugs.

The effect of any drug is related to the dose given, its bioavailability and the patient's ability to metabolize the drug.

Factors affecting drug function in children
Renal function
- The glomerular filtration rate is 10% of adult values in neonates and reaches adult levels by 1 year of age.
- Renal tubular function matures by 6 months.
- There is a proportionally larger extracellular fluid compartment, so some drugs, such as suxamethonium, need to be given in higher doses in small infants and neonates.
- Renal enzyme systems mature at different rates.

Immaturity of the receptors
- Maturation of enzyme systems, particularly in the renal, hepatic and immune systems, takes place at varying rates and is often unpredictable.
- Once systems are mature, metabolism may be more rapid than in the adult because of the high metabolic rate and good tissue perfusion of the child.

Integrity of the blood–brain barrier (BBB)
- The BBB matures over the first few months of life. In neonates, the BBB is more permeable than in adults and drugs cross more easily. This is particularly common in premature babies.
- The integrity of the BBB can be affected by hypoxia or sepsis.

Differences in absorption through the gut
- The effect of a drug may be altered by changes in pH, which affects the ionization of the drug. Gastric acid secretion is decreased in neonates.
- Stomach emptying and gut motility may be depressed.
- Drugs given rectally may have an unpredictable effect, the amount absorbed depending on:
  - type of preparation given
  - dose given
  - the degree of first-pass effect.
- There is a variable degree of metabolism of drugs within the bowel wall.
- Differences in distribution.

Protein binding
There is less protein binding of drugs in neonates because there is:

- Decreased plasma protein values, particularly albumin.
- Lower levels of α_1-acid glycoprotein. This is particularly important for binding local anaesthetics. Normal values are reached by about 6 months.

With less drug bound to protein, the amount of unbound drug increases. It is this unbound fraction which is active. For example, lignocaine has half the protein binding in neonates as in adults, hence doses must be decreased to ensure blood concentrations remain below potentially toxic values.

Regional tissue perfusion
The rate of absorption will be affected by the perfusion at the site of administration. This varies in children because:

- The relative blood flow to various organs is different in neonates than older patients.
- In comparison to adults, the percentage of cardiac output going to the kidneys and muscle is considerably lower in neonates.
- Because the neonatal brain is proportionally larger than the adult brain, it receives a greater portion of the cardiac output – 25%. This is one reason why induction agents act more quickly in the very young.

Muscle
- Babies have a low muscle mass.
- Receptors at the neuromuscular junction may be immature, or there may be a decreased number of receptors in the very young.

Fat stores
- Lipid soluble drugs are stored in fat. In the infant, only 10% of the body composition is fat. This rises to 30% at 1 year and then decreases.

Liver function
- Metabolic rate is higher in the young, so drug clearance may be more rapid.
- Impaired circulation with decreased liver blood flow will affect the metabolism and clearance of those drugs which rely on hepatic function.
- Enzyme systems may be immature. The P450 enzyme system has low activity in neonates, increasing to peak activity in early childhood, and reaching adult levels by puberty. The immaturity of the enzyme systems affects many processes including the excretion of drugs, the efficacy of the first-pass effect and the ability to induce enzyme systems.

Induction agents
In general, smaller doses are used in neonates (see Box 2.1).

Box 2.1   Doses of induction agents in paediatrics

Agent	Dose
Propofol	2–5 mg/kg
Thiopentone	3–7 mg/kg, (2 mg/kg in neonates)
Ketamine	IV 1–2 mg/kg
	IM 10 mg/kg
Etomidate	300 µg/kg

Propofol
- Increasingly popular for induction in children.
- Widely used for induction of anaesthesia in children aged less than 3 years, but not licensed for use in children of this age group.
- Infusions are not recommended in paediatric practice. There have been reports of fatal cardiac failure in intensive care children who were treated with propofol infusions. The high-risk group appears to be those with respiratory infections but, because of safety concerns, propofol is not used for routine maintenance of anaesthesia.
- Infants require higher induction doses than children.
- There may be some rare circumstances (e.g. anaesthesia for children with malignant hyperthermia) where infusions of propofol are appropriate.

Side effects
- Greater decrease in blood pressure than thiopentone.
- Decreases systemic vascular resistance (SVR).
- Bradycardia common especially < 2 years.
- Dose-related apnoea.
- Pain on injection 20–40%, decreased with addition of lignocaine, (1 mg for each 10 mg of propofol).

Thiopentone
- Redistribution is rapid.
- Action is prolonged in neonates as clearance is delayed, because of enzyme immaturity and low plasma protein levels.
- Recovery is slower than with propofol.
- Less effect on blood pressure than propofol.
- Less apnoea.
- Does not cause pain on injection.

Ketamine
- Remains popular in paediatrics especially for short procedures and investigations, e.g. bone marrow sampling, X-ray procedures.
- Can be given IV, IM, orally.
- Has dissociative side effects such as nightmares and disorientation, so benzodiazepines should be given. The incidence of these complicates in young children is difficult to quantify.
- Reduced clearance in neonates due to immature liver metabolism.
- Provides some analgesia.

- Less respiratory depression, laryngeal reflexes preserved.
- Blood pressure well maintained, has a role in cardiac anaesthesia.

Inhalational agents
General considerations in paediatrics
Gaseous induction remains very popular in paediatric practice. It is frequently the induction method chosen by older children. Sevoflurane has become the induction agent of choice although halothane is also used.

The requirements of an ideal inhalational induction agent for paediatric use include:

- pleasant odour
- non-irritant
- safe, non-toxic, non-explosive
- rapid onset and recovery, i.e. low blood/gas partition coefficient
- low MAC and high potency, high oil/gas partition coefficient
- minimal cardio-respiratory depression
- analgesia
- controllable muscle relaxation.

Minimum alveolar concentration (MAC)
The MAC of most agents is lower in the neonate, increases to a maximum 50% above adult values at about 6 months, and decreases to approximately adult values before puberty (see Box 2.2).

Box 2.2   MAC of inhalational agents in different age groups

	< 6 months	< 1 yr	Adult
Halothane	0.8	1.2	0.75
Sevoflurane	3.1	2.5	1.7
Isoflurane	1.6	1.8	1.15
Desflurane	8	11	6.0

In comparison with adults, uptake is quicker and is inversely related to age so that this effect is more marked in the younger child. This is due to:

- increased alveolar ventilation
- lower blood gas solubility and tissue blood solubility due to the different proportions of body water, fat and protein

- more rapid distribution especially to vessel-rich group
- more rapid elimination.

There is decreased solubility and decreased metabolism of inhalational agents in young paediatric patients. This may partly explain why inhalation-induced hepatitis, 'halothane hepatitis', is so uncommon in paediatric practice.

Specific inhalational agents
Halothane (see Box 2.3)
Internationally, the most widely used inhalational agent in children.

Box 2.3   Advantages and disadvantages of halothane use in children

Advantages	Disadvantages
Cheap	Slower than sevoflurane
Safe	Pungent smell
Depresses laryngeal reflexes, excellent for laryngoscopy, ENT procedures and management of the difficult airway	Atrial and ventricular arrthythmias common, especially ventricular extrasystoles
	Dose-related hypotension, decreased cardiac output due to decreased contractility
	Sensitizes the myocardium to exogenous adrenaline (epinephrine)
	Rarely associated with hepatitis
	Dose-related increase in cerebral blood flow and intracranial pressure

---

Halothane hepatitis
- Hepatitis has been reported with *all* inhalational agents but mostly with halothane.
- Very rare, < 1 in 200 000 halothane anaesthetics.
- Many children have had multiple halothane anaesthetics uneventfully.
- Less drug is metabolized in children so less metabolite is present.
- Associated with halothane-induced antibodies.

Sevoflurane
- An expensive agent which has gained popularity for gaseous induction in children.

- Well-tolerated, non-irritant with an acceptable smell.
- Cardiovascular stability with little effect on heart rate.
- Dose-related apnoea.
- Similar side effect profile to halothane (cough, laryngospasm, desaturation, secretions) at induction and emergence.
- Emergence delirium. Effective analgesia must precede recovery from anaesthesia. Delirium may occur in the absence of pain; e.g. after magnetic resonance imaging, the incidence is 30%.

Metabolites of sevoflurane
- 5% of sevoflurane is metabolized by hepatic cytochrome P450 enzymes: 20% halothane, 0.2% isoflurane and 0.02% desflurane.
- Metabolites include free fluoride ions. Levels > 50 mmol/l are toxic in adults, but not reached in children.
- Little likelihood of renal toxicity.
- Compound A (which causes renal damage in rats) is produced during the passage of sevoflurane through soda lime. Although, theoretically, there is potential for toxicity, this has not been reported either experimentally or clinically.

Isoflurane
- This agent is more pungent than halothane and is associated with more airway irritation at induction.
- Excellent agent for maintenance of anaesthesia, with few cardiorespiratory effects.
- Less cardiovascular depression than halothane.
- Some decrease in heart rate.
- Little effect on cerebral blood flow, useful for neurosurgery.
- Less metabolism than halothane.
- Recovery is quicker than halothane.

Desflurane
- Not popular for gaseous induction as it is associated with airway irritation, cough and laryngospasm.
- Strong, pungent smell.
- Expensive.
- Little effect on cerebral blood flow.
- Good maintenance agent with rapid recovery.
- Increases heart rate due to sympathetic stimulation.

Premedication

Atropine

This is used less frequently preoperatively as IV induction agents have gained in popularity. The pre-induction placement of an IV cannula allows IV administration in the few patients that require it. It is occasionally used preoperatively as a vagolytic and drying agent.

Particularly useful:

- Before ENT procedures, as it causes decreased secretions and so fewer airway complications at induction or emergence. Topical lignocaine before micro-laryngoscopy and bronchoscopy is more effective when atropine has been given, as it results is better mucosal contact of the lignocaine.
- For the management of the difficult paediatric airway, before fibre-optic intubation.
- In neurosurgery (controversial).
- In infants.

Usually oral atropine is given, but occasionally it is administered IV or IM as the bioavailability of oral atropine is unpredictable.

Midazolam

- Highly lipid soluble and passes through the BBB rapidly.
- Metabolized in the liver. Some metabolites are weakly active, they are glucuronidated, and excreted in the urine.
- Used orally in children.
- Dose-related side effects including sedation, ataxia, double vision, and respiratory depression.
- Can be given nasally.
- Action antagonized by flumazenil.
- Dose of 0.5 mg/kg orally is associated with minimal side effects, predictable anxiolysis within 30 min and no delay in discharge.
- When used as an infusion in the very young, the binding sites may become saturated, and with diminished excretion, accumulation occurs.

Other uses:

- When compared with adults, the half-life is considerably longer in the neonate and less so in the infant (90 min in children and 5 h in neonates).
- Clearance is much lower in neonates.

Chloralhydrate, triclofos

Both are metabolized to trichloroethanol but triclofos is a more pleasant mixture. It is a very effective, reliable sedative, but has a longer onset and offset time than midazolam.

Muscle relaxants (See Box 2.4.)
Suxamethonium

The duration of action is similar to adults. With a fast onset, it is used for rapid sequence induction in all age groups.

- A larger dose is required in neonates and infants, 1.5–2 mg/kg, because the distribution volume is greater.
- Neonates may have decreased activity at the neuromuscular junction receptors.
- Bradycardia is common.
- Hyperkalaemia can occur in children with burns, paraplegia, muscular dystrophies or myopathy.
- Mild myoglobinuria is common in children.
- Can be used effectively IM.

Non-depolarizing agents

- Neonates and infants are more sensitive to these drugs than older children and adults.
- Their duration of action is longer, probably because of immaturity of muscle fibres and receptor sites, which mature over the first 3 months.
- There is a higher volume of distribution.
- Delayed elimination.

Mivacurium

- Metabolized by plasma cholinesterases.
- Larger doses required, often twice the adult dose.
- Action is shorter in children for single dose and infusions.
- Can cause histamine release.

Atracurium

Smaller doses in infants and larger doses in children has been reported, but this is not important clinically.

- Metabolism by Hoffmann elimination.
- No accumulation.

- Volume of distribution and clearance rate is greater in infants.
- Minimal effect on the cardiovascular system.
- Histamine release increases with age but rarely important.

Cisatracurium
- A more potent isomer of atracurium. Its duration is longer than atracurium, but it has similar pharmacology.
- Cleared faster in children than adults.
- Does not produce histamine release or cardiovascular changes.

Rocuronium
- Has a faster onset, produces a more profound motor block, and lasts longer in infants than in older children.
- Clearance slower in infants and highest in children (because of differences in volume of distribution) then decreasing to adults levels. Duration of block is shortest in children.
- Increasing the dose decreases the onset time, making it a useful drug for modified rapid sequence induction in young children.
- Can be used IM.
- Metabolized in the liver, and to a lesser extent by the kidney.

Vecuronium
- Action is prolonged in infants.
- Smaller dose in infants, highest at 4 years as children have faster clearance than babies or adults.
- Associated with mild tachycardia.
- Mainly hepatic metabolism excreted in bile.

Box 2.4   Dose schedules for muscle relaxants in children

Muscle relaxant	Intubating dose (µg/kg IV)	Infusion rate
Suxamethonium	1.5–2.0	
Mivacurium	0.3	
Atracurium	0.5	6 mcg kg/min
Cisatracurium	0.1	
Rocuronium	0.6	
Vecuronium	0.08–0.10	1.5 mcg kg/min (use half this in neonates)
Pancuronium	0.1	

Pancuronium

- Long acting.
- Vagolytic, associated with tachycardia, which is well tolerated in children.
- Used in cardiac anaesthesia.
- Excretion mainly by kidney, delayed excretion in neonates.

Reversal agents

Neuromuscular monitoring is essential and if adequate return of function is present, reversal is not always necessary.

Neostigmine, dose 25–50 µg/kg, lower doses in infants. This is given with atropine 20–25 µg/kg, or glycopyrolate 10 µg/kg.

Analgesics

Opiates

- Babies are liable to the side effects of morphine, particularly respiratory depression and sedation, and these are more common in small babies.
- Active metabolites of morphine accumulate, as liver enzymes involved in glucuronidation are slow to mature. Clearance is erratic until 3 months of age.
- Infusions of morphine need to be carefully monitored. Neonates may require postoperative respiratory support if they have received fentanyl during anaesthesia.
- Fentanyl is much more lipophilic and it therefore has a large apparent volume of distribution. It is cleared slowly by liver metabolism; its action is prolonged and is unpredictable in infants aged less than 6 months.
- Epidural opiates are avoided in small infants, as transfer of morphine across the BBB is variable.
- Babies and children probably suffer from nausea, vomiting and pruritis but it is difficult in these age groups to ascertain the prevalence of these complications.
- Bradycardia and hypotension occur with all opiates and are dose-dependent.
- Chest wall rigidity, 'wooden chest' can occur with opiates, particularly fentanyl.
- Alfentanil has a similar side-effect profile to fentanyl. Metabolism relies on the hepatic cytochrome P450 enzyme system, which is greatly reduced in activity in neonates.
- Remifentanil, which is metabolized by tissue cholinesterases, avoids the problems of hepatic or renal immaturity. It has a shorter and more predictable half-life.

- Codeine is still widely used in paediatrics. It has less respiratory depression, is effective orally, IM and rectally. It is metabolized to morphine. A single dose is safe in self-ventilating neonates, though repetitive dosing can lead to accumulation. The analgesic efficacy of codeine is very variable due to genetic variants of enzyme systems.

Paracetamol

- Hepatic metabolism of paracetamol in neonates is as effective as in adults. In the neonate, more of the drug undergoes sulfonidation which is an effective process, and little undergoes glucuronidation, which is immature.
- Absorption and excretion can be slower in neonates. In neonates the maximum oral dose in **24h** is 60 mg/kg and in older patients 90 mg/kg.
- Some studies use very large loading doses, but the daily dose limit should be adhered to. Reversible liver toxicity occurs rarely with normal dosage regimens.
- Doses needed for an antipyretic effect are lower than those required for analgesic effect.
- The absorption of paracetamol given rectally is less predictable.

Non-steroidal anti-inflammatory drugs (NSAIDs)

- Main drugs in use are diclofenac and ibuprofen.
- Used, in combination with paracetamol, to treat mild to moderate pain.
- Care needed if platelet function or number is decreased.
- Generally, there is no measurable change in pulmonary function in children with mild to moderate asthma when NSAIDs are used.
- Avoid in patients with abnormal renal function.
- Not used in neonates and small babies because of decreased renal blood flow.

Local anaesthetics

Most work has been done with lignocaine and bupivacaine, particularly looking at plasma values after caudal injections, or in neonates following maternal epidurals.

In neonates and young infants:

- There is rapid absorption of local anaesthetics due to high tissue blood flow and cardiac output.
- The metabolism of local anaesthetics is decreased because of immature enzymes systems.

- The volume of distribution is higher and the half-life is prolonged.
- Plasma proteins levels, especially α_1-acid glycoprotein, are low, therefore protein binding is less.
- High plasma levels may be reached and so toxicity increased.
- The use of infusions (e.g. epidurals) is associated with an increased likelihood of side effects, especially in the very young.

3

Equipment and monitoring in paediatric anaesthesia

Equipment for use in paediatric anaesthesia has changed in recent years and the quality of equipment available now is unrecognizable from even 10 years ago.

Ideal characteristics of a paediatric breathing system
- low resistance
- no valves
- small dead space
- lightweight
- ability to provide continuous positive airways pressure (CPAP)
- universal connections.

Paediatric breathing systems
Ayre's T piece
The most commonly used circuit in paediatric anaesthesia is the Mapleson F circuit, the Jackson Rees modification of the Ayre's T piece (the addition of an open-ended bag and increased length of the inspiratory limb). It has most of the ideal characteristics of a paediatric breathing system (see above).

Features of the Ayre's T piece are
- Suitable for both spontaneous and controlled ventilation.
- Used in patients weighing up to 15–20 kg
- End-tidal CO_2 concentrations are determined by fresh gas flow and minute ventilation.
- Can be used with a ventilator such as the Penlon ventilator with paediatric Newton valve (Fig. 3.1).
- Easy to scavenge anaesthetic gases from the end of the inspiratory limb using a specially designed device.

Fresh gas flow

Various formulae have been used to determine the fresh gas flow required to prevent rebreathing with this circuit during spontaneous and controlled ventilation. The flows required to prevent rebreathing are high. However, in practice, some rebreathing is an advantage as heat, moisture and anaesthetic gases are preserved and pollution and costs are reduced. With the advent of reliable capnography, these formulae are less important as fresh gas flow is determined by the end-tidal CO_2 level.

The Bain circuit

Features of the Bain circuit are:

- It is a coaxial T piece with fresh gas delivered to the patient along the inner tube, and exhaled gas vented through the outer tube.
- Useful in patients > 20 kg.
- Suitable for spontaneous and controlled ventilation.
- The circuit can be long because the fresh gas is always delivered at the patient end of the circuit.
- A valve is present at the proximal end of the circuit.
- Easy to scavenge anaesthetic gases.
- End-tidal CO_2 concentrations determined by a combination of fresh gas flow and minute ventilation.

Circle system

The semi-closed circle system which incorporates soda lime for CO_2 absorption is now used widely in paediatric anaesthesia (see Box 3.1). The adult circuit is adapted by using smaller diameter tubing and a ventilator capable of ventilating small children. There is now a wide variety of suitable ventilators for use with this circuit.

Box 3.1   Advantages and disadvantages of the circle system

Advantages	Disadvantages
Economic as less anaesthetic agent is used	Increased resistance so may not be ideal in small infants breathing spontaneously
Reduced pollution	
Conservation of heat and moisture	Valves can stick
	Cost of soda lime

Ventilators

In the simplest terms, ventilators are classified as either pressure generators or flow generators. Flow generators provide a predetermined inspiratory tidal volume while pressure generators produce a predetermined inspiratory pressure. Flow generators compensate for increases in compliance such as in asthma, whereas pressure generators compensate for leaks in the circuit but not changes in compliance.

Pressure-controlled ventilation is commonly used in paediatric anaesthesia because there is often a leak around the endotracheal tube and because there is risk of barotrauma.

The ideal characteristics of a paediatric anaesthetic ventilator are:

- Good ergonomics and simplicity of use.
- Provision of volume- and pressure-controlled ventilation.
- Provision of variable positive end expiratory pressure (PEEP).
- Compatible with a circle system.
- Variable I : E ratio.
- Built in alarms including:
  - high pressure
  - oxygen concentration
  - expired tidal and minute volume
  - disconnect.
- Easy to change from controlled to manual ventilation without changing circuits.
- Ability to generate very small tidal volumes for use in neonates.

Many current ventilators have most of the above features.

The Penlon Nuffield 200 ventilator

The Penlon ventilator is still widely used in paediatric anaesthesia. The Penlon is gas powered and, with the adult patient valve connected, operates as a flow generator. The inspiratory flow rate is set in ml/sec. The inspiratory volume is determined by a combination of the inspiratory time and the inspiratory flow rate. In adults or in children weighing more than 20 kg it is used in conjunction with the Bain circuit.

In children < 20 kg, the adult patient valve is removed and a paediatric Newton valve is attached (Fig. 3.1). This valve changes the Penlon from a flow generator to a pressure generator and the flow rate selected on the ventilator is not the flow rate delivered to the patient.

The Newton valve is simply a fixed orifice which allows some of the selected inspiratory flow to go to the patient while the remainder is

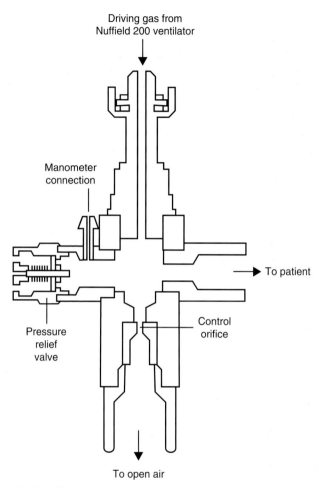

Driving gas from
Nuffield 200 ventilator

Manometer
connection

To patient

Pressure
relief
valve

Control
orifice

To open air

Figure 3.1 The Newton valve.

vented through the fixed orifice. The pressure generated is shown by the pressure indicator on the ventilator.

It is essential that a disconnect (pressure) monitor is used with a Penlon ventilator. The use of an expired gas volume alarm has also been recommended.

Special Note: Before connecting a child to the Penlon ventilator, the end of the Ayre's T piece should be occluded and the pressure generated noted. This will prevent the possibility of barotrauma if the adult valve has been inadvertently connected.

Box 3.2   Advantages and disadvantages of Penlon ventilator

Advantages	Disadvantages
Inexpensive	No inbuilt alarms
Easy to use	Risk of barotrauma if adult valve is inadvertently used in patients under 20 kg
Simple robust design	
Compatible with Ayre's T piece and Bain circuit	Uses large volumes of driving gas
Reliable	Sound of ventilator remains unchanged with disconnection and occlusion of breathing system
	Pressures remain unchanged with occlusion of breathing system
	Inadvertent PEEP applied when patients > 15 kg ventilated with Ayre's T piece
	Patients between 15 and 20 kg may be too small for adult valve and too large for paediatric valve
	Difficult to provide active humidification

Paediatric anaesthesia masks

Face masks are used for:

- Preoxygenation before rapid sequence induction.
- Inhalational induction.
- Spontaneous ventilation during anaesthesia.
- Positive-pressure ventilation before intubation.

Ideal characteristics include:

- Small dead space.
- A good fit to the face.
- Made of clear plastic. This makes them more acceptable to children and allows the colour of the lips and the presence of vomit to be observed.
- Non-latex.
- Soft rim to prevent trauma.

Many masks are also available with various scents such as strawberry or raspberry.

There are specially designed face masks to allow fibreoptic intubation. These have the connector for the fresh gas flow attached to the side of the mask. There is a small self-sealing aperture in the centre of the mask to allow the passage of the fibreoptic bronchoscope. Alternatively, an ordinary face mask can be used with an angle piece which allows the passage of the bronchoscope through a self-sealing aperture.

Airways
Oropharangeal airways
The Guedel oropharangeal airway comes in a wide variety of sizes from 000–3 and larger for adults (see Box 3.3). Sizing the airway is done by holding an airway along the child's mandible from the mouth. The airway should ideally reach from the mouth to the angle of the mandible.

Box 3.3   Sizes of oropharangeal airway in children

Age	Size
Preterm	000–00
Neonate–3 months	0
3–12 months	1
1–5 yr	2
> 5 yr	3

Nasopharangeal airways
- Not usually used during routine anaesthesia.
- Better tolerated than an oral airway because they do not produce such a strong gag reflex.
- May be used if the child has sleep apnoea, or other upper airway obstruction, and requires support O_2 postoperatively.
- Possible to use CPAP with nasopharangeal airways.

Nasal airways are made from very soft rubber with a flange at the end to help hold them in place. Alternatively, they can be made from an endotracheal tube one size smaller than would be used for intubation and cut short. The length should be measured from the nose to the external auditory meatus.

The laryngeal mask airway (LMA™)
The development of the LMA™ has been a major advance in paediatric anaesthesia. A range of paediatric sizes has ensured that the LMA™ has become a routine part of airway management (see Box 3.4).

Features of the LMA™:

- The LMA™ is designed to sit with the tip at the upper oesophageal sphincter, the sides in the pyriform fossa and the upper portion at the base of the tongue.
- It is made largely of silicone, is latex free and consists of a tube connected to a spoon-shaped mask with an inflatable rim. The rim is inflated through a pilot tube which is sprung loaded to keep the rim inflated.
- An magnetic resonance imaging-compatible LMA™ (yellow pilot balloon) without a metal spring is available, which reduces image artifact.
- A non-kinking LMA™ is available. This is slightly awkward to insert because the tube is not rigid.
- The LMA™ is reusable for a maximum of 40 times.
- It is sterilized with the cuff deflated after gentle washing by autoclaving for 4–5 min at not more than 134°C. Each mask should have its own card which records the number of cycles it has undergone.
- The masks come in seven sizes from 1 to 5. Sizes 1–3 are used in children.

Box 3.4   Sizes of LMAs™ used in children

Size	Weight (kg)	Cuff volume (ml)
1	< 5	2–4
1½	5–10	4–6
2	10–20	10
2½	20–30	14
3	> 30	25

Insertion of the LMA™ requires an adequate depth of anaesthesia using inhalational anaesthesia or IV propofol. Thiopentone and the other agents do not provide good conditions for insertion of the mask unless anaesthesia is deepened with volatile agents before insertion. The insertion technique varies between anaesthetists. After lubrication of the mask, some will insert the LMA™ deflated and inflate the cuff once it is in position. Others (including the author) prefer to insert the mask with it either fully, or partially, inflated. The main obstacle to insertion in children comes from the relatively large size of the tonsils. To facilitate easier insertion, the mask is advanced until the resistance of the tonsils is felt and then turned 90° and advanced to its final position.

The LMA™ is generally used for spontaneously breathing patients, but it can also be used for positive-pressure ventilation.

Gastric distension with intermittent positive-pressure ventilation is much less likely if inflation pressures are < 20 cmH$_2$O. This practice is not widely used and great care must be taken not to inflate the stomach. The LMA™ does not protect against aspiration of regurgitated gastric contents and is contraindicated in those at risk of aspiration.

The LMA™ has a particular role in the paediatric difficult airway. It can be used not only to secure an open airway in patients in whom it is difficult to hold a mask, for example patients with Hurlers syndrome, but it can also be used to enable fibreoptic intubation in cases of difficult intubation, for example in Pierre–Robin syndrome.

Tracheal tubes and intubation
Size of tracheal tubes

The narrowest portion of the trachea in small children is at the level of the circular cricoid ring and not the vocal cords. It is easy to provoke tracheal oedema, or more importantly permanent subglottic stenosis, by trauma at intubation. It is important to use the correct size of tracheal tube in infants and neonates (see Box 3.5 and 3.6). The most reliable method is to ensure that the tracheal tube passes the glottis and cricoid ring without resistance, and that a small leak can be heard at an inspired pressure of 20 cmH$_2$O.

In children older than 1 year the following formulae are used:

- size of tube (mm) = $\dfrac{\text{age}}{4} + 4$

- the length of the oral tube (cm) = 3.5 × internal diameter (mm).

Box 3.5   Tracheal tube sizes and length in neonates

Weight (kg)	Tube size (ID) (mm)	Oral length (cm)
0.7–1.0	2.5	7.0–7.5
1.0–1.5	2.5	7.5–8.0
1.5–2.0	3.0	8.0–8.5
2.0–2.5	3.0	8.5–9.0
2.5–3.0	3.0	9.0–10.0
3.0–3.5	3.5	10.0–10.5

Box 3.6   Tracheal tube sizes in the first year of life

Age	Usual weight (kg)	Tube size (mm)	Length (cm)
Newborn	3.5 kg	3.5	10–10.5
6 months	6.5 kg	4.0	11.5–12.5
1 year	10 kg	4.5	13–13.5

It should be remembered that all information about the size and length of tubes is only a guide and that great care must be taken that the tracheal tube selected is not only the correct diameter but also the correct length. Most tracheal tubes are marked in centimetres. This enables the anaesthetist to place an exact length through the cords. There is in addition a black line running along the tube to indicate how far the tube should be advanced through the cords.

Correct tracheal length can ensured by various methods including:

- Observing the length of tube through the cords.
- Advancing the tube until the right main stem bronchus is entered (by ausculating the left chest) and then withdrawing the tube into the trachea.
- Equal bilateral breath sounds.
- Equal bilateral chest movement.

Types of tracheal tube

There are a wide range of tracheal tubes available for use in children. Most are made of implant-tested PVC although some are made from silastic or even metal.

These include:

- PVC tracheal tube.
- Preformed south-facing polar tubes (RAE, invented by Ring, Adair and Elwyn). These tubes are occasionally too long when the correct size is selected and have a hole at the distal end of the tube (Murphy's eye) to ventilate the right upper lobe if this occurs.
- Preformed north-facing polar nasal tubes.
- Armoured or non-kinking silastic tubes.
- Cole tube. A shouldered tube with the distal end narrower than the rest of the tube. The intention of this design was for the narrow part of the tube to go through the vocal cords, with the shoulder coming to rest on

the cords, preventing endobronchial intubation. These tubes are seldom used in anaesthesia because of potential damage to the cords.
- Metal laser tubes.
- Cuffed tubes are available even in the smallest sizes.

The use of cuffed tubes in children
It has been traditional teaching that non-cuffed tracheal tubes should be used in small children and this is certainly a safe practice. However, there are some anaesthetists who advocate the use of cuffed tubes even in small infants.

The use of cuffed tubes may reduce trauma to the trachea because the contact with the mucosal surface is by a soft, low-pressure, high-volume cuff, rather than by the rigid surface of the uncuffed tube. In addition, cuffed tubes may avoid the potential for multiple intubations if the first tube selected is not the correct size. Generally, it is necessary to select half a size smaller than would be chosen for a plain tube.

Laryngoscopes
The large, floppy epiglottis and more cephalad position of the laryngeal inlet in infants means that intubation is easier using a straight-bladed laryngoscope. In smaller infants less than about 6 months of age the technique of intubation is different from that with older children and adults. The straight blade is used to lift the epiglottis directly to reveal the laryngeal inlet.

A number of different laryngoscope blades are available for use in paediatric anaesthesia. Common straight-blade laryngoscopes include:

- Anderson–Magill
- Seward
- Robertshaw
- Miller.

These blades vary in longitudinal and cross-sectional shape.

Temperature measurement and warming devices
Effects of hypothermia
The preservation of core body temperature is important in paediatric surgery. In general, the reduction in body temperature is associated with increased morbidity.

Morbidity includes:

- increased oxygen consumption by:
  - shivering in children
  - non-shivering thermogenesis in neonates
- increased sympathetic stimulation
- reduced immunity
- delayed wound healing
- patient discomfort
- reduced platelet function
- impaired coagulation
- increased blood loss and transfusion requirement
- reduced drug metabolism
- myocardial depression
- cerebral depression
- acidosis
- possible cardiac shunt reversal
- delayed discharge from recovery.

Heat loss

Initially, after induction of anaesthesia heat is redistributed to the periphery because of vasodilation. This results in a rapid fall in core temperature of about 1°C. Subsequently, loss of temperature slows to about 0.5°C per hour.

Heat loss in the operating room occurs by:

- radiation – 50%
- convection – 30% (if uncovered)
- evaporation from skin, respiratory tract and open body cavities. More significant if patient is wet.
- conduction – least significant

Temperature measurement

It is very important to measure temperature in all children undergoing surgery. This is not only to prevent hypothermia but also to prevent hyperthermia if any active heating device is used.

Temperature is measured using:

- Thermistors and thermocouples – most commonly used for continuous intraoperative monitoring of core temperature.
- Liquid crystal thermometers – used for skin temperature.

- Infrared thermometers – used for atraumatic, tympanic temperature measurement.

Core temperature can be measured at a number of sites:

- Nasopharyngeal – approximates to brain temperature but may be low because of cooling from a large leak around the tracheal tube.
- Oesophageal – this more accurately reflects core temperature if the distal third of the oesophagus is used. The proximal oesophagus may be cooled by gases from the tracheal tube.
- Rectal – may be inaccurate and changes slowly if faeces are present.
- Tympanic membrane – accurate reflection of core temperature. Infrared atraumatic tympanic probes are required.
- Bladder.

The purpose of measuring skin temperature is to monitor the difference between core and peripheral temperature to give information about peripheral perfusion.

Maintaining temperature
Covering
The proportion of total body surface area covered is important; the head of infants is relatively large and therefore a major source of heat loss.

Ambient temperature
The neutral thermal environment is the ambient temperature at which there is no increased oxygen consumption to maintain body temperature. The smaller and younger the infant, the higher the temperature required, which makes the working environment uncomfortable.

Heated mattress
These may be electric, warm water or warm air. They are not particularly efficient.

Warm air blowers
Disposable over- or under-blankets are used with these devices. The blankets are designed to circulate warm air around the patient and are very effective.

Overhead radiant heaters
These are effective, and portable models are available. They should always be used with the skin probe provided so as not to overheat the

skin. These heaters are particularly useful in the anaesthetic area while the patient is uncovered.

Warmed and humidified inspired gases
This is usually achieved passively by:

- a heat and moisture exchanger
- partial rebreathing with Ayre's T piece
- use of circle system.

Warmed fluids and blood products.

Monitoring
The same standards of monitoring used in adults also apply to children. Monitors should be placed before induction of anaesthesia and remain until the patient has recovered. In paediatric anaesthesia, it is occasionally difficult to apply monitors to children who are very upset and it is sometimes better to induce anaesthesia and then apply the monitors.

Electrocardiogram (ECG)
- The ECG is a good monitor of heart rate, rhythm and changes in configuration of the complexes.
- The monitor must be able to filter unwanted electrical noise.
- Lead II is most commonly monitored for rhythm changes.
- S-T changes may be due to ischaemia, pericarditis, myocarditis or electrolyte disturbance.
- Placing the leads on the limbs rather than the chest is a good alternative in children.

Pulse oximetry
- The pulse oximeter detects hypoxaemia in children. It is less effective in detecting hyperoxia.
- The presence of foetal haemoglobin does not alter the accuracy of the pulse oximeter in children. Also, it is accurate over a wide range of haemoglobin concentrations.
- It is important to maintain the oxygen saturations of premature infants in the range 90–95% to reduce the risk of retinopathy of prematurity.
- Response times vary depending on where the probe is placed. The buccal mucosa and ear lobes may produce the fastest response times.
- Paediatric probes are available which can be wrapped around a finger, toe, hand or foot.

- Accuracy may be lost with severe anaemia, polycythemia, methaemoglobinaemia, and carboxyhaemaglobinaemia.

Capnography

Capnography provides information about:

- adequacy of ventilation
- pulmonary blood flow
- cardiac output
- airway dynamics:
  - bronchospasm
  - kinked tracheal tube
  - leak around tracheal tube
- rebreathing
- state of neuromuscular blockade
- patient breathing against ventilator.

The accuracy of capnography in children may be affected by:

- Dilution by high fresh gas flows if a partial rebreathing system is used.
- Use in very small babies with low tidal volumes and high respiratory rates.
- If a large leak is present, the plateau of the capnograph does not occur. If PEEP is also present, the trace may be lost completely.
- Cyanotic congenital heart disease: the $ETCO_2$ underestimates the arterial CO_2 and the worse the cyanosis, the greater the difference between arterial CO_2 and $ETCO_2$.

Two types of capnograph are available:

- In-line analysis: this is more common in adult practice because the sampling device is large and heavy and thus unsuitable in paediatrics.
- Side-stream analysis: this is most commonly used in paediatric anaesthesia. A small amount of inspired and expired gas is constantly withdrawn from the breathing system for measurement.

Anaesthetic agents and oxygen concentrations are also measured from the same sampling port in integrated monitoring systems.

Non-invasive blood pressure measurement

It is now possible to measure blood pressure accurately even in small premature infants. This is done usually using the oscillometric technique.

Many different sizes of cuffs are available, with five neonatal sizes alone. It is important to select the correct size cuff. Too small a cuff will produce an abnormally high reading and too large a cuff will produce an abnormally low value.

In full-term, normal-sized neonates, a cuff width of 4 cm is used. In older children, the cuff width should be approximately 40% of the arm circumference for optimal accuracy.

Invasive blood pressure measurement

Invasive blood pressure measurement is required when:

- major surgery is undertaken
- cardiovascular instability is expected
- blood sampling is required (blood gases, electrolytes and haematocrit)
- major blood losses are anticipated.

Invasive pressure monitoring provides useful information about the cardiovascular status of the patient. A trace which alters with positive-pressure ventilation usually indicates hypovolaemia, while a sharp narrow trace (small area under the curve) usually indicates a reduced cardiac output. In both examples, the blood pressure may be nearly normal.

Complications of intra-arterial monitoring include:

- occlusion or thrombosis of vessel with distal ischaemia
- infection
- haematoma
- embolization
- necrotizing enterocolitis from cannulation of umbilical artery.

The risk of embolization can be reduced by not re-injecting aspirated blood, and by flushing the cannula with small volumes of fluid at low pressure.

The radial artery is most commonly used, other arteries include the femoral, axillary, ulnar, dorsalis pedis and, occasionally, the brachial artery.

Central venous pressure (CVP) monitoring

The indications for CVP monitoring in paediatric anaesthesia are similar to those for arterial monitoring. In addition, the need for infusions of inotropes or other potent drugs may require the placement of a CVP catheter.

The CVP, which approximates to the right atrial pressure, reflects the relationship between right-sided filling pressure, right heart function and peripheral vascular resistance. It is a useful measurement but the response to a fluid bolus is more useful than absolute values alone.

Common sites for central venous access include:

- internal jugular vein
- subclavian vein
- femoral vein.

After cardiac surgery, direct placement of catheters in the left or right atrium, pulmonary artery, is sometimes required.

Complications of CVP line placement include:

- accidental arterial puncture
- pneumothorax
- air embolism
- infection
- vessel erosion
- thrombosis and embolism
- bacterial endocarditis.

The use of heparin-bonded catheters reduces the incidence of infection and thrombosis in children with central venous lines.

Neuromuscular monitoring

It is important to use peripheral nerve stimulation when neuromuscular blocking drugs are given.

Nerves used include:

- Ulnar nerve, on the medial aspect of the wrist or in the ulnar groove at the elbow.
- Posterior tibial nerve, behind the medial malleolus.
- Facial nerve.
- Posterior tibial nerve at the head of the fibula.

Heart and breath sounds

Heart and breath sounds can be monitored using either a precordial or oesophageal stethoscope. Although this type of monitoring is not commonly used in the United Kingdom, it is frequently used in the USA.

Heart sounds can give information about:

- heart rate and rhythm
- cardiac output
- presence of air in the heart (machine room murmur).

Breath sounds can monitor:

- ventilation
- bronchospasm.

4

Anaesthesia for the infant and child

Infancy is the time between the end of the neonatal period and 1 year of age. The neonatal period is defined as the first 28 days of life. Specific issues are discussed in the specialist chapters and general principles of paediatric anaesthesia are addressed here.

Preoperative preparation

The anaesthetist will see the child preoperatively and discuss the plans for anaesthesia. Books, videos or ward visits all help in preparation.

The play specialist is an important member of the team. When giving information to children, it is important that it is appropriate for the child's level of understanding. Young children need to be given information a few days before the event, whilst older children can remember and digest information given in the weeks preceding surgery.

The preoperative visit is useful to the child, their family and to the anaesthetist because it ensures that:

- The child is ready for theatre.
- All investigations are satisfactory.
- The child and family have been fully informed about the planned procedure and their opinion has been sought regarding the options for the anaesthetic, particularly that the choice of an inhalational or IV induction has been explained and their preference sought.
- The anaesthetic plan is agreed and consent is taken (usually verbal).
- Documentation is complete.

Anxiety is common in children and many children find it difficult to express their worries. Usually, parents are present at induction and on recovery, which is helpful for the child and the parent. A program of psychological preparation can help children with severe anxiety or phobias, e.g. related to theatres or needles.

Consent

The options for anaesthesia, and the risks and benefits of the alternatives, must be fully discussed with the parent/person with parental responsibility. Any specific techniques, such as need for blood products, use of a local block, use of suppositories, use of arterial or central venous cannulae, likelihood of admission to an intensive care unit, or any specific risks, should be discussed. Consent is usually given by a parent or legal guardian for a child.

Children over the age of 16 years are deemed competent to give consent themselves. Children, of any age, who are deemed able to understand the implications of having or refusing surgery and considered 'Gillick competent' can give consent. However, patients aged less than 16 years can refuse care, but the courts at present support parents and doctors who consent to operating 'in the best interests of the child'.

The child who is unable to cooperate

Some children are acutely anxious, or may have learning difficulties, so it unrealistic to expect them to cooperate with induction of anaesthesia. This has to be handled sensitively considering the legal regulations on consent for procedures. With the support of the parent, adequate premedication and gentle encouragement, most children accept induction of anaesthesia.

It may be helpful to give sedation the night before surgery, e.g. temazepam. On the day of surgery, oral midazolam up to 1 to 1.25 mg/kg has been used safely for premedication, although the incidence of side effects such as diplopia, blurred vision and unsteadiness increases with this increased dose. Intranasal midazolam is effective but not popular, especially with older children, as it tends to irritate the nose. Oral ketamine is sometimes helpful and IM ketamine is occasionally used. Placement of an IV cannula on the ward can smooth the induction period considerably.

Risk

The risk of complications during anaesthesia increases with increasing ASA status. For ASA I & II children, the risk of a serious complication is less than 1 in 10 000; the risk for neonates is higher, approximately 40 per 10 000.

Fasting

Excessive periods of fasting do not enhance stomach emptying and are unpleasant for the child. Fasting can occasionally result in dehydration and hypoglycaemia, particularly in small infants. Prolonged fasting also increases the use of IV fluids, adding potential risks and cost. All children should stop taking food 6 h preoperatively, but the provision of clear fluids until 2 h preoperatively results in a gastric volume and pH that are similar to those found in children who have been starved for ≥ 6 h. Clinically significant aspiration of gastric contents is uncommon in paediatric anaesthetic practice, it is usually associated with difficulties in airway management.

The prevalence of aspiration is 1 in 9000 to 1 in 25 000. Small babies frequently aspirate small amounts of their milk feeds and seem to tolerate this. Children who do aspirate are frequently asymptomatic and, if they have no symptoms or signs 2 h after aspiration, are unlikely to develop pulmonary problems.

The management of clinically significant aspiration includes continued ventilation, supportive therapy, physiotherapy and antibiotic treatment. This usually results in rapid recovery.

Fasting guidelines for elective surgery
Clear fluids can be given until 2 h preoperatively:

- No breast milk for 4 h.
- No formula milk for 6 h.
- No food for 6 h.
- Most regular medication can be given in the preoperative period but this is dependent on individual drug regimens.
- The relevance of carbonated drinks or chewing gum remains controversial.

Investigations
These must be relevant to the medical condition of the child and the planned surgery.

Healthy children do not require preoperative blood tests. Screening, for haemoglobinopathies such as haemoglobin S, is done in any patient at risk.

The normal haemoglobin value depends on the child's age (see Box 4.1). Studies of elective day-stay children have shown that anaemia is uncommon and when present it is almost always due to dietary iron deficiency. Whether a child with mild anaemia is postponed, investigated and treated, or allowed to proceed with anaesthesia, does not affect the perioperative outcome. Haemoglobin concentration should be measured in any child with a clinical reason to suspect anaemia and in any child who may

Box 4.1 Haemoglobin values and age	
Age	Hb (g/dl)
Preterm	17
Term baby	17.8
3 weeks	15
6–12 weeks	9.5–11
2–10 years	11–13

require transfusion as a result of the surgery, to provide a baseline from which to monitor and assess blood loss and replacement.

Small children have a relatively small circulating blood volume and may require transfusion after modest losses. Therefore, children need to have their blood 'grouped and saved' or cross-matched for procedures that would not require this in adult practice. This includes most laparotomies, cleft palate surgery, and closure of colostomy. Transfusion is avoided wherever possible and peroperative haemoglobin estimations ensure blood is only given when necessary.

Premedication

The need for premedication is related to the child's physical and psychological state and the requirements of anaesthesia for the particular surgery. Most children do not require premedication, but no patient should be barred from the potential benefits of carefully chosen preoperative medication on the basis of ward policies. There are many different drugs available and many routes of administration have been used. Commonly used sedative drugs include midazolam, temazepam or triclofos. Other drugs include:

- Ametop (amethocaine gel 4%, tetracaine), which can be used in term babies above 1 month. Use is occasionally associated with sensitivity resulting in reddening of the skin and sometimes weal formation. There are isolated reports of severe reactions. It is effective for several hours. EMLA is licensed above 1 year, but used extensively in younger patients.
- Atropine, which has an antisialogogue and antivagolytic effect. It is frequently used in airway surgery and in small infants before a gaseous induction. Its use is controversial and unwanted tachycardia can occur. If the use of topical local anaesthesia of the airway is planned, the decrease in secretions following atropine allows effective action of locally applied lignocaine. In small babies, the cardiac output

is rate dependent and bradycardia is poorly tolerated, so the vagolytic effect of atropine is useful during gaseous inductions, to antagonize the negative inotropic effect of many inhalational agents.

Childhood infections

In general, it is unwise to undertake elective anaesthesia during the course of an acute infection. Viral upper respiratory tract infection (URTI) is one of the most common illnesses in children, who have an estimated 2–9 episodes of URTI per year. Other infections such as viral gastroenteritis, chickenpox, measles or rubella pose a potential risk to the child because of increased morbidity such as lower respiratory tract infections with chickenpox. In addition, many children in hospital will be immunocompromised and must be protected from the infected child. All hospitals have a policy on the control of infection to avoid local spread and minimize the risk of hospital acquired infection.

Upper respiratory tract infection (URTI)

There is conflicting evidence on whether there is increased risk when a child has an URTI. Some studies of day case children have shown up to an 11-fold increase in perioperative complications including cough, laryngospasm, bronchospasm, oxygen desaturation and stridor. This is probably the result of increased sensitivity of the airways, increased airway secretions, and an increased tendency for small airways to close during anaesthesia. Complications were greatest in young children and infants, and in those who required tracheal intubation. Other work has suggested that the rate of complications is little changed in the presence of a mild URTI.

Major morbidity and even mortality (from myocarditis or pulmonary collapse) has been reported in children with URTI who have undergone anaesthesia, but these reports are sporadic.

It is wise to postpone children who have a fever > 37.5°C, who are miserable, anorexic, coughing, wheezing, or have chest signs. The more difficult group is those that are relatively well but have mild nasal discharge, or a slight temperature, but no other signs or symptoms. Many children who would have had no problems may be cancelled.

The following factors have been shown to help in making a decision:

- signs and symptoms
- temperature
- white blood cell count
- chest X-ray

- parental concerns
- Age (< 1 year have increased complications).

Monitoring standards

All patients should be monitored from the start of anaesthesia to the end of recovery. Some paediatric patients cannot tolerate external monitors before induction but these should be placed when consciousness is lost.

Routine monitoring includes:

- electrocardiogram (ECG), non-invasive blood pressure, SPO_2, plethysmography
- FiO_2
- capnography, anaesthetic vapour analyser
- temperature
- neuromuscular function.

Perioperative fluid management

Many children will not require IV fluids perioperatively provided they have had clear fluids up to 3–4 h before the procedure and are likely to be drinking adequately after surgery.

When calculating the fluid needs of the paediatric patient take into account:

- the length of preoperative fasting and the likelihood of the child drinking after surgery.
- intraoperative losses
- maintenance requirements
- third space and evaporative losses
- blood loss
- postoperative fluid requirements (maintenance fluids + losses).

A child's fluid status is assessed clinically (see Box 4.2).

Calculating fluid requirements
Preoperative deficit
If the preoperative fast has been longer than 4–6 h consider replacing the deficit. This is calculated as follows:

- Preoperative deficit = hourly fluid requirements × length of fast (h).
- This amount is transfused during surgery if there is sufficient time, otherwise the fluid can be given postoperatively.

Box 4.2 Assessment of dehydration

Degree of dehydration % body weight	Sign/symptom
5%	Tachycardia
	Dry mucous membranes
	Decreased urine output
10%	Loss of skin turgor
	Oliguria
	Sunken eyes
	Sunken fontanelle
15%	Tachycardia
	Decreased blood pressure
	Slow capillary refill
	Poor peripheral perfusion, cool extremities
	Acidosis

Hourly maintenance

Many different formulae are used to calculate fluid requirements (see Box 4.3). One simple method is:

- 4 ml/kg/h for the first 10 kg
- 2 ml/kg/h for the second 10 kg
- 1 ml/kg/h for the remaining weight.

Box 4.3 Fluid maintenance formulae

Weight (kg)	Volume (ml/kg/h)
< 10	4
10–20	2
> 20	1

Example

A 32 kg child requires 72 ml/h for full replacement. (10 kg @ 4 ml/kg/h + 10 kg @ 2 ml/kg/h + 12 kg @ 1 ml/kg/h (*40 + 20 + 12*))

However:

- Fluids are often restricted for the first postoperative day to half the maintenance amount, as fluid retention is likely.

- Fluid choice is dictated by clinical requirements, see below.
- In the sick child, fluid resuscitation should be done before anaesthesia.
- Any additional losses must be added to the hourly maintenance.

Choice of IV fluids
Crystalloid
Initial requirements are met with a crystalloid infusion. During surgery a balanced solution, Hartmann's solution, is used outside the neonatal period. If a bolus of fluid is required, 10–20 ml is given and the effect assessed.

Small babies may need additional glucose and solutions containing 10% or 20% dextrose may be given. The amount is dictated by the blood glucose values. Care must be taken not to give large volumes of hypotonic solutions to children; isotonic solutions should be used. In theatre, fluid is given using a burette or chamber system so that volumes are measured accurately. Postoperative fluids are usually given via volumetric pumps for accurate rate of administration. Measurements of serum electrolytes and glucose must be done regularly if IV fluid regimens are continued postoperatively and 2–3 mmol K^+ are added to each 100 ml of fluid if the serum K^+ is low.

Colloids
Used for volume replacement.

Gelatins, hydroxyethyl starches
Albumin is now used less commonly due to concerns about safety. There are worries about potential transmission of prion disease. It is used mostly in neonates as either a 5% or 20% solution and may be associated with increased mortality.

Blood and blood products
- Used only when essential. The level of haemoglobin, which requires blood replacement, varies depending on the child's condition and on local policies. It is usual to permit haemoglobin values of 7 g/dl in the otherwise well child before considering transfusion.
- There are increasing concerns with the risk of transfer of infection.

Blood requirements can be estimated in various ways:

- Intravascular volume status is best assessed clinically. This includes pulse rate, blood pressure, peripheral perfusion, core–peripheral temperature gradient, urine output, central venous pressure and acid–base status.

- Haemoglobin or haematocrit values ensure accurate use of red blood cells.
- Measure blood loss (this can be difficult and inaccurate in practice). Clinical parameters are the best guide.

One useful method in determining the amount of replacement blood is to use haematocrit levels:

$$\text{Blood required} = \frac{\text{Hct1} - \text{Hct2}}{\text{Hct3}} \times \text{EBV}$$

Hct1 = haematocrit before transfusion, the measured haematocrit.
Hct2 = haematocrit required after transfusion, the desired haematocrit.
Hct3 = haematocrit of the blood to be given (60% if packed cells).
EBV = estimated blood volume.

This equation can be used to estimate the volume of blood that could be lost before transfusion. It also allows measurement of the amount of blood required to replace losses and achieve a designated haemoglobin.

An alternative method is to use the formula:

$$(\text{Hct1} - \text{Hct2}) \times \text{Body weight (kg)} \times 1.5 = \text{volume of packed red cells}$$
$$\times 2.5 = \text{volume of whole blood}$$

Hct1 = measured haematocrit.
Hct2 is the desired haematocrit.

The need for other products such as platelets, cryoprecipitate or fresh frozen plasma (FFP) should be guided by coagulation studies.

- Platelets and FFP are usually only given if the haematology screen or clotting studies show significant deficit.
- If the platelet count is low < 50–80 000, 5–10 ml/kg platelet infusion is given.
- FFP is given as a 10–20 ml/kg infusion to provide coagulation factors.
- Cryoprecipitate may be needed if disseminated intravascular coagulation is present or fibrinogen levels are low.

Recovery

Many children are comfortable breathing on an LMA™ until awake. However, laryngeal reflexes are more pronounced in the younger age groups and coughing or laryngospasm may occur during recovery. In small children, therefore, we advocate removal of the LMA™ at a deep plane of anaesthesia.

All patients who have had muscle relaxants should have their neuromuscular function measured. They may not require reversal of neuromuscular blockade if there is adequate return of function as indicated by:

- Double-burst stimulation producing two equal contractions.
- Sustained contraction with tetanic stimulus at 50 Hz.
- Return of a regular, effective respiratory pattern.

Following extubation of the trachea, children transferred from the operating theatre to the recovery area require:

- presence of the anaesthetist
- oxygen by face mask
- placed in a lateral position unless contraindicated by surgery
- some will require monitoring with ECG, SpO_2 during transfer.

In recovery, monitoring includes:

- respiratory rate and pattern
- blood pressure, heart rate, oxygen saturation
- temperature
- level of consciousness
- assessment and management of:
  - pain
  - postoperative nausea and vomiting (PONV)
  - blood loss
  - fluid balance

Complications in recovery
- Complications are more common in younger patients: 7–10% in children 1–12 years and 7–15 % < 1 year. The frequency of critical incidents after surgery is related to the ASA status of the child.
- Postoperative complications may cause delayed discharge or unplanned overnight admission.

Complications include
- Respiratory:
  - decreased O_2 saturation (mixed aetiology)
  - laryngospasm
  - stridor
  - airway obstruction.

- Cardiovascular:
  - blood pressure/heart rate changes
  - bleeding/post surgical complications.
- Emergence delirium, occasionally an effect of midazolam or sevoflurane.
- Excess sedation, delayed discharge.
- PONV occurs in approximately 20% of patients. Risk factors include:
  - ENT, eye surgery – up to 50–80%
  - abdominal surgery
  - opiate use
  - long procedures
  - age (commoner in older children, probably under-reported in the young who are less distressed by it).

Antiemetics used in children include cyclizine, metoclopramide or ondansetron.

Hypothermia

Particularly important in small babies, those at risk from hypothermia should be transferred immediately to a heated incubator and may need to be nursed in a high-dependency area.

Children are discharged from recovery when they are:

- awake
- maintaining their airway
- normothermic and have a stable cardiovascular system
- comfortable and any complications have been dealt with.

Late effects of surgery

Frequently families are not aware of what to expect in the early postoperative period. They may be reluctant to provide regular analgesia and need to be given patient advice.

Complications such as pain, PONV and behavioural changes may persist. These may be due to the surgery, anaesthetic or the perioperative process. It is useful if all children are reviewed after surgery and these effects managed actively. Behavioural changes such as poor sleeping, nightmares or personality changes are quite common, although the aetiology is unclear. Such changes may take 4–6 weeks to resolve.

Pain management
Good pain management is essential in paediatrics:

- Pre-emptive analgesia is useful.
- Combination of local blocks and systemic analgesia improves pain management.
- Clear guidelines are essential for the assessment and management of postoperative pain and any complications.

There are several pain scoring systems available including:

- CHEOPS (Children's Hospital of Eastern Ontario Pain Scale).
- Objective Pain Scale.
- Faces scale.

Further reading
Recommendations for Standards of Monitoring during Anaesthesia and Recovery. December 2000, The Association of Anaesthetists of Great Britain and Ireland. Available: http://www.aagbi.org.

5

Paediatric day care

Guidelines from the Royal College of Surgeons suggest that 50–70% of elective paediatric operations should be done as day cases.

Successful day care requires careful selection and screening of appropriate patients, use of an efficient system of care with an expert multidisciplinary team, good analgesia protocols and effective postoperative follow-up.

Advantages of day care
- shorter hospital stay/quicker return home
- less emotional upset
- less parental separation
- fewer behavioural problems (such as alternation to sleeping pattern, nightmares, enuresis, regression)
- less likelihood of acquiring a hospital-based complication such as infection
- improved parent satisfaction
- improved child satisfaction
- decreased cost
- decreased waiting lists
- increased turnover and use of resources
- release of resources for inpatient care.

Disadvantages of day care
The increased workload can increase costs. In addition, more care may be moved into the community, management of pain or postoperative complications, and this needs to be well organized and resourced.

Common day-care procedures include
- Inguinal or femoral hernia repair
- Orchidopexy
- Umbilical hernia repair
- Circumcision
- Suture removal
- Grommet insertion
- Adenoidectomy
- Otoplasty
- Dental extractions and conservations

- Bone marrow aspirates
- Lumbar punctures
- Insertion of indwelling venous lines
- Radiological scans
- Squint surgery
- Eye examinations
- Changes of plaster
- Removal of metalwork

Requirements for a paediatric day-care service
- multidisciplinary approach
- dedicated team members
- well-designed unit
- good support in the community.

Quality standards for paediatric day care
The National Association for the Welfare of Children in Hospital report in 1991 outlined standards for paediatric day care. Their document, 'Just for the Day', had the following recommendations:

1. A day-care plan should be integrated to include pre-admission, day of admission and post-admission care with a planned transfer of care to the community.
2. The child and parent should be prepared before and during the day of admission.
3. Specific written information should be given to parents.
4. Children should be admitted to dedicated day-care areas and not mixed with acutely ill inpatients.
5. Children should not be admitted or treated alongside adults.
6. Specifically designated day staff should care for the child.
7. Only staff with paediatric and day-care experience should manage the child.
8. Care should be organized so that every child is likely to be discharged within the day.
9. The building, equipment and furnishings should comply with children's safety standards.
10. The environment should be child friendly.
11. Essential documentation should be completed before the child's discharge to ensure efficient after-care and follow-up.
12. There should be paediatric nursing support available for the child at home.

Design of a paediatric day-care unit
The above criteria should be taken into account when designing a new unit. Ideally, a paediatric day unit should have separate areas for the

different age groups, e.g. babies, toddlers, teenagers. A good design aims to allow the child to progress through the unit, to theatres and recovery areas, without pre- and postoperative patients mixing. Most efficient units will have designated day-care theatres next to the unit. Paediatric day-care facilities should also include the following:

- reception area
- waiting area
- playroom
- office space
- clinic rooms for history taking and examination
- clinical room for taking blood
- locker space for clothes
- toilet and shower facilities
- the bed or trolley area will need to have piped gases, suction and the ability to include monitoring equipment if required
- small kitchen
- storage facilities
- staff facilities
- independent unit with good links to hospital support services
- all should be child friendly and with easy access.

Contraindications to day care
The individual child must be considered in terms of his/her medical condition and the proposed surgery.

Medical or surgical
- Prolonged surgery (duration of surgery up to 1 h only, though this is not applied rigidly).
- Surgery associated with significant pain or bleeding post operatively.
- Emergency surgery.
- Children needing specialized preoperative care, e.g. diabetes, metabolic disease.
- Acute illness such as upper respiratory tract infection, respiratory syncytial virus, chickenpox, gastroenteritis.
- Malignant hyperthermia.
- Latex allergy.
- Haemophilia, significant bleeding disorders.
- Sickle cell disease.
- Complex cardiac disorders.
- Projected airway difficulties, sleep apnoea.
- Neonates and babies < 60 weeks' postgestational age.

Social
- Reluctance to be a day case.
- Inadequate family support.
- Long distance to travel.
- Lack of adequate transport.
- No telephone.

Babies
The age at which babies are suitable for day care depends on all the above criteria. Many units use 6 months as the lower age limit for term babies but some units will provide day care to term babies over 4 weeks of age. Preterm babies and expremature babies (born before 37 weeks' gestation) are at increased risk of postoperative apnoea and bradycardia. These babies must be monitored with an apnoea alarm and SpO_2 measurement on the postoperative night, so should not be treated as day cases. The age at which an expremature baby is no longer at risk from these sequelae is unclear, but is probably 56–60 weeks postgestational age.

Preoperative preparation, investigations and premedication

Preoperative preparation
Effective day care requires streamlined assessment. Protocols for fasting and investigations should be clear and given to the parent before admission. Preoperative information about the child may be collected at a preoperative screening clinic, by telephone, or on the day of surgery.

Questionnaires are very useful for screening suitable patients for day care. Preoperative clinics, which are nurse led and include input from the surgeon, anaesthetist and the play specialist, are increasingly common and very effective. These assessment clinics are associated with improved parent satisfaction, less stress in the parent and child, a decrease in late cancellations and more effective use of resources and time. On the day of surgery, the child and family are reviewed by the surgical and anaesthetic teams undertaking their care.

Psychological preparation
Clear explanation of the procedure and the anaesthetic is very useful. Preoperative play therapy, videos, booklets and discussions are all helpful.

Investigations
Most children require no preoperative investigations. Routine haemoglobin estimation has been shown to be unnecessary in ASA I and II

day patients and should be confined to children with a history indicative of a potential abnormality such as previous anaemia or known blood dyscrasias. A sickle screen is necessary in children who may have sickle cell anaemia. Otherwise, investigations are dictated by the physical condition.

Premedication

Premedication is often unnecessary in day cases but is not contraindicated and should be considered for each child. Oral midazolam 0.5 mg/kg is not associated with delayed recovery and is well tolerated if sedative premedication is required. Oral atropine 20 µg/kg may be necessary for small children, particularly those requiring airway surgery. Antiemetics and analgesics are useful, particularly in older children and those having eye or dental surgery. EMLA or Ametop is used if an IV induction is planned.

Anaesthesia

Parents are usually encouraged to be present at induction. The child often makes the choice of either intravenous or inhalational induction. Intravenous induction is with either thiopentone or propofol. Propofol, although not licensed for children aged under 3 years, is widely used and has become very popular, particularly in the older child. Thiopentone has not been shown to delay discharge. Large doses of propofol 4–5 mg/kg, are required if the LMA™ is inserted immediately. If a smaller dose of propofol is used, anaesthesia can subsequently be deepened with inhalational agents to allow insertion of an LMA™. Sevoflurane is the commonest induction agent in children. It is well tolerated and has rapid onset. The side effects at induction are similar to halothane. After inhalational induction, an IV cannula is always inserted. The LMA™ is used extensively in paediatric day surgery, but intubation is not contraindicated. Maintenance anaesthesia is usually with isoflurane O_2/N_2O. Opiates may be given as required, but care must be taken as the incidence of postoperative nausea and vomiting, and the likelihood of delayed recovery, increase with repeated doses. Intravenous fentanyl, morphine and IM or rectal codeine phosphate can be used.

Good postoperative analgesia is essential for successful day-case surgery. Whenever possible, regional analgesia or local infiltration should be used in combination with general anaesthesia. The addition of paracetamol and non-steroidal anti-inflammatory drugs started in theatre and continued postoperatively improves the quality of the analgesia. Intravenous fluids are not required routinely as children should not be fasted for long periods preoperatively and most day surgery is short and not associated with significant fluid losses. However, IV fluids can be useful particularly in children with an increased risk of postoperative nausea and vomiting (PONV), those that have been fasted extensively preoperatively, and in small infants. The use of perioperative fluids, together with allowing children to go home without drinking before discharge, is associated with lower levels of PONV.

Local anaesthetic techniques suitable for day cases include infiltration, caudal block, ilioinguinal block, axillary block, penile block, infraorbital block, and greater auricular nerve block. They provide several hours of analgesia. The use of adjuncts, such as opiates, is contraindicated in day-case patients due to the risk of side effects such as respiratory depression. Clonidine has been used as an additive in caudal blocks although there is additional sedation and a risk of transient hypotension.

Recovery

Children usually recover quickly and can be discharged rapidly. Suitable discharge criteria include:

- Return to consciousness and age-appropriate activity. Older children may need to be able to walk.
- Stable vital signs.
- Minimal or no nausea or vomiting.
- Adequate pain control and appropriate analgesia for postoperative use.
- Surgical site is dry with no active bleeding.
- No surgical complications.
- No serious anaesthetic problems.
- Postoperative information has been given and is understood. This includes details of the surgery, anticipated sequelae, instructions for the management of pain, when to start eating and who to call with any postoperative query.
- Clear instructions for follow-up must be given. Some units telephone each family on the day after surgery; others have a member of the community nursing team who visits each child after surgery.

Audit

Useful outcome measures, which should be continuously audited, include:

- reasons for cancellation
- non-attendance
- pain
- fasting times
- vomiting
- anaesthetic complications, surgical complications
- unexpected admission
- delayed discharge
- readmission rate
- readmission reason.

6

Anaesthesia in the neonate

Definitions
- A neonate is a baby aged up to 28 days.
- A premature baby is born before 37 completed weeks, postconception. Thus, the age of a baby is referred to as the number of weeks postconceptional age (PCA) or post-gestational age (PGA).
- A term baby is born 37–40 weeks' PGA and those 42–44 weeks' PGA are referred to as postmature.

Therefore an expremature baby may be 3 months old (a baby born at 28 weeks PGA and aged 12 weeks) may just have reached its expected date for delivery – 40 weeks' PGA. Premature and expremature babies have special risk factors associated with anaesthesia. All babies should be anaesthetised in centres which have the resources and expertise to care for them throughout the perioperative period.

Preoperative assessment and premedication
Preoperative assessment of the neonate includes
- age and maturity
- weight
- general physical condition
- associated congenital abnormalities
- investigations
- vitamin K.

Postgestational age and weight
A healthy term baby born between 37 and 42 weeks usually weighs 2.5–3 kg. Babies tend to lose weight over the first week of life and then start to gain weight. This effect is more pronounced in premature babies. Babies may be small for dates, premature or both. Very low birth weight babies are defined as < 1500 g, and extremely low birth weight < 1000 g. Survival in tiny babies has improved with expert neonatal care; however, mortality and the incidence of complications in survivors increases with decreasing birth weight.

Babies who are large for gestational age may have:

- increased risk of birth trauma
- risk of hypoglycaemia, increased feeding required
- polycythaemia.

The most common cause of babies being large for gestational age is maternal diabetes. Other causes include babies with transposition of the great vessels, those with Beckwith–Wiedemann syndrome and those born post-term.

Premedication

Neonates do not usually require sedation. Atropine, can be given when required, either orally or, less frequently, IM. It is used for vagolytic activity and to decrease airway secretions. Atropine may also be given IV on induction, either routinely, or if bradycardia occurs.

Ametop can be used as a local anaesthetic cream to assist IV cannulation. EMLA is not recommended for babies < 12 months old as metabolism of prilocaine may produce methaemoglobinaemia.

Investigations

Haemoglobin

All neonates should have a haemoglobin estimation before surgery as the concentration is related to the degree of foetal/maternal transfusion at birth and is therefore unpredictable (see Box 6.1). Babies who have been in hospital for prolonged periods are frequently anaemic because of:

- disease
- difficulties with establishing adequate feeding
- repeated blood sampling.

Anaemia is associated with an increased incidence of apnoea postoperatively, particularly in the premature neonate.

Box 6.1	Normal neonatal haematological values	
	Birth Mean (range)	1 month Mean (range)
Haemoglobin	18 (14.5–21) g/dl	14 (10–16) g/dl
White count	5–25	6–15
Reticulocytes	3–7%	0–1%

Sickle cell disease testing

At birth, the main form of haemoglobin is fetal haemoglobin (HbF). This is gradually replaced, in the first 3 months of life, by adult forms of haemoglobin, usually haemoglobin A (HbA).

In patients with sickle cell disease (SCD) HbF is replaced by haemoglobin S rather than HbA so that by about 3 months significant amounts of HbS are present.

Initially, babies with SCD are protected from the effects of abnormal haemoglobin by the high HbF concentration. This means that Sickledex screening may provide false negatives in a very young baby with sickle cell disease, as HbS levels are so low. However, electrophoresis will be accurate in this age group as it identifies all haemoglobin types present. Many babies at risk from SCD can be screened using cord blood and this is routinely done in many centres.

Bilirubin

Neonates are frequently jaundiced; 80% of preterm babies and 50% of term babies have jaundice. There are many causes, but jaundice until 4 weeks of age can be physiological. Jaundice may be due in part to relative polycythaemia at birth and the immature hepatic enzymes that are unable to deal with the additional red cell load. Physiological jaundice is due to increased unconjugated bilirubin values. If conjugated bilirubin is raised, then other causes must be sought. Physiological jaundice may be treated with phototherapy or exchange transfusion, as unconjugated bilirubin can cross the immature blood–brain barrier and cause brain damage (kernicterus).

Other investigations are dictated by the baby's physical condition. Clotting studies are often required, as neonates are at risk from coagulation factor deficiencies due to:

- immaturity of the coagulation system
- presence of sepsis, frequently associated with thrombocytopenia and coagulopathy
- jaundice
- vitamin K deficiency.

Vitamin K

Vitamin K is necessary for production of hepatic coagulation factors II, IV, IX and X. It is given routinely at birth to prevent haemorrhagic disease of the newborn. Vitamin K is given either IM as a single injection or as a course of three oral doses. The anaesthetist should ensure that Vitamin K has been given before surgery.

Induction and maintenance of anaesthesia

Sevoflurane is the inhalational induction agent of choice in most neonates. It has a rapid onset with cardiovascular stability. Thiopentone remains a useful agent, but propofol is unlicenced in this age group and there is little information about this agent in neonates. Ketamine is used occasionally.

For all but the shortest procedures, neonates require tracheal intubation and ventilation. This is because the functional residual capacity is reduced so that closing volumes are near to tidal volumes leading to the risk of ventilation/perfusion mismatch.

It is necessary to minimize apparatus dead space. Whilst the size 1 LMA™ provides a convenient airway it is liable to dislodgement and longer procedures are poorly tolerated due to the small degree of respiratory reserve in neonates.

Atracurium is the most useful muscle relaxant as neonatal enzyme systems are immature with unpredictable metabolism of other relaxant drugs.

Maintenance of anaesthesia is with oxygen in either nitrous oxide or air. It is important to avoid administration of excessive concentrations of oxygen in premature babies.

A nasogastric tube is used as abdominal distension inhibits lung expansion and ventilation may be compromised.

Management of temperature

Small babies loose heat quickly and have poorly developed physiological mechanisms for maintaining body heat.

Measures used to aid thermal care

- Always monitor temperature.
- Maintain a warm thermal environment, increase theatre temperature.
- Use active warming, e.g. an overhead radiant heater.
- Transfer in an incubator.
- Warm inspired gases or use a heat–moisture exchanger.
- Heat conservation-wrap exposed areas using foil, bubble plastic or cotton gamgee.
- Use warm air mattress.
- Warm IV fluids.

Analgesia

Historically, neonates were thought not to feel pain but this has been disproved. Babies mount a significant hormonal stress response to surgery if they are not given sufficient anaesthesia or analgesia. It has been suggested that they have increased morbidity and mortality if anaesthesia is inadequate. It is often difficult to assess pain in the very young as their responses are different from older children.

Pain management during minor surgery is often provided by the combination of local anaesthesia (either as a block or as infiltration of the wound) and paracetamol. Following major surgery, pain management with epidurals or morphine infusions can be used in neonates providing the child can be monitored adequately in a high-dependency area.

Local anaesthetic
Blocks such as caudal or ilioinguinal are used commonly. It is often useful for the surgeon to inject the local anaesthetic by the ilioinguinal nerve under direct vision. Epidural (caudal or lumber) and spinal blocks have been used in neonates for many years.

The maximum safe dose of local anaesthetics is lower in neonates. Plain bupivacaine or ropivacaine are used for epidual analgesic. Opiates are avoided as they have an increased incidence of side effects, particularly respiratory depression.

Paracetamol
Paracetamol is used to a maximum dose of 60 mg/kg/day, orally or rectally.

Non-steroidal anti-inflammatory drugs (NSAIDs)
NSAIDs are not used for analgesia in this age group as the renal system is immature and their effect has not been extensively investigated.

Opiates
Codeine phosphate 1 mg/kg IM or rectally is useful after minor/moderate surgery and is safe provided it is not given IV. Particular care must be taken with the use of opiates in neonates. Morphine, fentanyl, alfentanil and remifentanil are all used. The incidence of complications, such as apnoea or respiratory depression is increased, particularly in babies < 5 kg. High-dependency care is required postoperatively if opiate infusions are used.

Fluid management
Fluid requirements can be divided into:

- Maintenance fluids, to cover the preoperative, perioperative and postoperative period.

- Third space and evaporative losses.
- Replacement of blood and clotting factors.

The fluid status of a baby is assessed using the following indicators:

- skin turgor
- peripheral perfusion, capillary refill time, e.g. of the finger tips
- fullness or sunken quality of the anterior fontanelle
- alterations in pulse and blood pressure
- haemoglobin and urea and electrolyte values
- estimation of insensible losses, for example, if the intestine is exposed the additional losses are approximately 5 ml/kg/h
- urine output (but this may be negligible on day one in the normal baby)
- knowledge of hourly requirements
- additional losses, e.g. blood, nasogastic fluid.

Routine maintenance fluid requirements in the newborn
- day 1 of life–2 ml/kg/h
- day 2–3 ml/kg/h
- day 3–4 ml/kg/h.

Maintenance fluid requirements on the first postoperative day are decreased to 2/3 of the usual daily amount.

Choice of fluid
- crystalloid – used for maintenance
- colloid – gelatin, albumin
- blood products.

Crystalloid
The choice of *maintenance* crystalloid fluid depends on the glucose and electrolyte needs. Usually 4% or 10% dextrose in 0.18% saline is used, with increased concentrations of dextrose if hypoglycaemia is likely. When losses from the gut are present, these are replaced with 0.9% saline with 10 mmol of potassium added to each 500 ml of fluid. This mixture is used to replace the hourly nasogastric volume on a millilitre for millilitre basis. These are guidelines only and fluid management requires careful monitoring of glucose and electrolyte values. The renal function of babies matures over the first few months. Neonates are not able to

excrete large volumes of water and may develop oedema easily. If an additional bolus of crystalloid is required it is usually given as IV saline or Hartmann's solution. Care must be taken not to administer excess crytalloid. Hypnotic solutions should not be used for volume replacement.

Hypoglycaemia

Neonates, and particularly premature or small for gestational age babies, are at risk perioperatively of hypoglycaemia, Although babies do have a glycaemic response to surgery due to surgical stress, they remain at risk of developing hypoglycaemia. It is important that small babies are provided with additional glucose, either by oral fluids or by infusion, if they are starved for long periods preoperatively. They may need additional 10% glucose infusion perioperatively. Term neonates can usually tolerate fasting according to standard guidelines. However, it is wise to measure blood glucose following induction of anaesthesia and treat hypoglycaemia if present with a bolus dose of 1–2 ml/kg of 10–15% dextrose.

Colloid

The use of albumin has become controversial after adult work linking its use with increased mortality in the intensive care unit. The relevance of this to neonates is unclear.

Other colloids such as the starch or gelatin solutions have not been extensively studied in neonates, but are used. There is concern that there may be accumulation of starch in the reticuloendothelial system of the neonate.

Blood

Perioperative blood losses must be closely monitored. Frequent determinations of haemoglobin allow accurate blood replacement. The aim is to achieve a normal neonatal Hb level by the end of surgery (see Box 6.1 above).

$$\text{Blood volume needed} = \frac{\text{Hct1} - \text{Hct2}}{\text{Hct3}} \times \text{EBV}$$

Hct1 = haematocrit before transfusion, the measured haematocrit.
Hct2 = haematocrit required after transfusion, the desired haematocrit.
Hct3 = haematocrit of the blood to be given (60% if packed cells).
EBV = estimated blood volume.

Sepsis in the neonate is frequently associated with thrombocytopenia and coagulopathy. Blood products such as fresh frozen plasma (FFP) and platelets may be required occasionally, especially in sick neonates undergoing major abdominal surgery. The use of these products should be guided by the results of a coagulation screen and full blood count.

Use of blood products in neonates
- Small babies tolerate blood loss poorly.
- It is usual to cross match blood for many procedures which would not require transfusion in older patients, such as formation of colostomy or insertion of Hickman line.
- Cross-matching blood has specific additional requirements in this age group:
  - Blood of the most recent donation should be used if large transfusion is required. Fresh whole blood contains clotting factors and active platelets so is very useful in sick neonates.
  - Blood must be filtered to remove white blood cells, which may transmit prion disease.
  - Babies with a presumptive diagnosis of DiGeorge syndrome require irradiated blood products.
  - Cytomegalovirus (CMV)-negative blood is used in neonates as their immune system is immature and CMV infection can be fatal.
  - FFP is used to replace clotting factors, (initially 10 ml/kg). This does not need cross-matching but is type specific; it must be given through a 150 µm filter.
  - Platelets are given only if the platelet count is low. Ideally, a single donor unit is used.

Fasting guidelines in neonates
- Breast milk may be given until 4 h preoperatively.
- Dextrose solutions may be given until 2 h preoperatively.
- Formula milk feeds may be given until 6 h preoperatively. These milks contain cow protein and are more slowly digested than breast milk.
- Babies having continuous feed via jejunal catheters should have these stopped 4 h preoperatively.

If surgery is delayed for extended periods, IV fluids must be given, or if time permits, additional clear oral fluids are given.

Monitoring

Routine monitoring should be used and is specifically designed for babies. This includes electrocardiogram, non-invasive blood pressure, FiO_2, E_tCO_2, anaesthetic agent, temperature, and neuromuscular function. As many neonates will have a patent ductus arteriosus the pulse oximeter should be placed on the right hand, if possible, to measure preductal SpO_2:

- E_tCO_2 monitoring is useful but the alveolar–arterial gradient may be considerable so that arterial CO_2 is poorly represented by E_tCO_2.
- In major cases, an arterial cannula is useful, usually in the radial, femoral or axillary artery.
- Central venous pressure is measured via the femoral or internal jugular vein.

Immediate postoperative management

At the end of surgery, most babies are extubated when awake and go to the recovery room. Neonates are not usually managed as day cases. Premature and expremature neonates will require additional monitoring for apnoea and bradycardia for at least the first 24 h postoperatively. Term neonates do not require this monitoring routinely. High-risk neonates, or those having extensive surgery, go to the neonatal unit and some will be electively ventilated postoperatively.

The premature and expremature baby

Babies born at less than 37 completed weeks of gestation are defined as preterm.

Conditions associated with prematurity include

- respiratory distress syndrome
- chronic lung disease
- bronchopulmonary dysplasia
- intraventricular haemorrhage
- visual or hearing loss
- retinopathy of prematurity
- increased incidence of congenital abnormalities
- necrotizing enterocolitis
- acquired subglottic stenosis
- persistent patent ductus arteriosus
- failure to thrive
- developmental delay
- cerebral palsy.

Retinopathy of prematurity

High PaO_2 in premature babies is associated with retrolental hyperplasia of the blood vessels, which may lead to retinopathy of prematurity and blindness. The aim is to keep the SpO_2 between 90% and 96%. The risk persists until about 8 months of age, and decreases with time, and the risk to an individual baby is difficult to estimate.

Postoperative apnoea

Apnoea is very common in preterm babies, and often associated with bradycardia. The risk is increased in premature babies following general anaesthesia or the use of sedation. Premature babies may have a history of apnoea which can be central, obstructive or mixed in aetiology.

Various definitions are used for postoperative apnoea, but a cessation of respiration for 15–20 sec, which may be associated with desaturation and bradycardia, is commonly used. These episodes are usually self-limiting or require mild stimulation of the baby to encourage respiration. Apnoea is more common in the more premature babies and occurs mainly in the first 24 h postoperatively.

Risk factors are:

- age less than 56–60 weeks PGA
- neurological disease
- anaemia
- general anaesthesia
- sedation
- opiate use
- known respiratory disease, e.g. bronchopulmonary dysplasia
- preoperative oxygen requirement.

Management

- Optimize condition preoperatively, e.g. treat anaemia.
- Monitor with a pulse oximeter and apnoea monitor for at least 24 h postoperatively.
- Consider use of caffeine pre- and postoperatively to decrease the risk of apnoea.
- Postpone routine surgery until after 60 weeks' PGA.
- Do not treat expremature babies as day cases until after 60 weeks' PGA.

7

Anaesthesia for general paediatric surgery

Many of the common conditions requiring surgery in young children are minor and can be undertaken on a day-care basis. Children are treated in most hospitals and frequently as part of mixed adult and paediatric lists, although dedicated paediatric lists are preferable. The principles of good paediatric care remain.

Appendicectomy

Appendicitis is the commonest cause of acute abdominal pain in children < 16 years (incidence 1 in 250).

Features

- Brief history of 1–2 days of symptoms, which includes pyrexia, abdominal pain, vomiting and occasionally diarrhoea.
- Some children present with peritonitis, and widespread sepsis can develop.
- Treatment is surgical, appendicectomy either by mini-laparotomy or laparoscopy.

Anaesthetic considerations

- Should be nil by mouth with a nasogastric tube in place, which should be aspirated before induction.
- Assume presence of delayed stomach emptying and plan a rapid sequence induction (RSI).
- IV maintenance fluids should be given preoperatively.
- Check full blood count (FBC) and U&E, as vomiting and sepsis may produce abnormalities.
- Group and save.
- Balanced anaesthetic technique with a RSI:
  - preoxygenation
  - cricoid pressure
  - IV induction with propofol or thiopentone

- suxamethonium
- tracheal intubation
- maintenance with O_2, N_2O and isoflurane/halothane or sevoflurane
- Fentanyl (1–3 µg/kg) or morphine (50–100 µg/kg).
- Postoperative analgesic management includes:
  - local infiltration of the wound
  - paracetamol, non-steroidal anti-inflammatory drugs (NSAIDs)
  - morphine infusion, either patient- or nurse-controlled analgesia depending on the ability of the child to use these techniques.

Intussusception

This occurs when one segment of bowel invaginates into a distal segment of bowel. This may result from a Meckel's diverticulum.

Features

- Commonly presents between 3 months to 3 years with a peak incidence at 6 months.
- Colicky abdominal pain, vomiting, passage of blood in the stool, 'redcurrant jelly stool'.
- Peritonitis with severe dehydration and electrolyte disturbance may develop.
- In the uncomplicated case, treatment may be with a barium enema, which reduces the invaginated bowel. If this fails, surgery is required with reduction of the intussusception or bowel resection.

Anaesthetic considerations

The anaesthetic requirements are those of a major laparotomy; surgery may be extensive:

- Considerable fluid resuscitation may be necessary before surgery. Some children are very sick and need to be treated in intensive care before surgery.
- Insert a nasogastric tube.
- Check the FBC, U&E, cross-match blood.
- Use a rapid sequence induction.
- Fentanyl or morphine.
- Most children can return to the ward; postoperative pain management is with a combination of IV morphine, NSAIDs and paracetamol.

- If the child is very sick, an arterial cannula, central venous catheter and urinary catheter are useful.
- Those children with sepsis, or with massive fluid loses, will require paediatric intensive care postoperatively and respiratory support.

Umbilical hernia

This is very common in babies, particularly premature infants.

Features
- usually asymptomatic
- most resolve spontaneously
- incarceration of bowel in the defect is uncommon
- repair is postponed until after 2 years if the hernia persists.

Anaesthetic considerations
- If the hernia is small, an LMA™ and spontaneous respiration is suitable; many are day cases.
- Larger hernias require abdominal muscle relaxation; therefore, tracheal intubation and ventilation are necessary.
- Local infiltration and simple analgesics are usually sufficient for pain management.

Nissans fundoplications

Gastro-oesophageal reflux is a common problem, particularly in children with muscular incoordination, e.g. cerebral palsy or severe developmental delay. Nissans fundoplication tightens the muscle at the gastro-oesophageal junction, reducing reflux and accidental aspiration of gastric contents. Surgery can be done via a laparotomy, using an upper transverse abdominal incision, or laparoscopically. Surgery is undertaken in all paediatric age groups.

Anaesthetic considerations
- Many children have recurrent chest infections, lung damage and poor respiratory function; their condition must be optimized.
- Pre- and postoperative chest physiotherapy is important.
- Poor nutrition is common; gastric bleeding may have been present. Preoperative FBC and U&E are essential.
- Blood is tested for 'group and save' as later cross-match and transfusion is occasionally required.
- Analgesic requirements depend on the type of surgery. With open surgery, an epidural provides efficient analgesia, preserves good

respiratory function and allows effective chest physiotherapy post-operatively. After laparoscopic surgery, only simple analgesics, short-term morphine infusions and local infiltration are required in most children.

- Morphine infusions are also effective. Care must be taken in monitoring side effects, such as sedation or respiratory depression, as many children have respiratory or neurological difficulties.

Laparoscopic surgery

Laparoscopic surgery is used increasingly in paediatric practice. Examples of procedures now done using the laparoscope include appendicectomy, inguinal hernia repair, Nissans fundoplication, splenectomy and colectomy. In general, laparoscopic surgery is considered less invasive and recovery is quicker. However, the procedures themselves are often prolonged.

Anaesthetic considerations

- Careful positioning is crucial to provide good conditions for any 'minimal access' surgery. Patients are usually supine and the position of the surgeon and the monitoring equipment is important and needs to be discussed with the surgeon.
- Distension of the abdomen with intra-abdominal gas, e.g. CO_2, and the use of a 'head-down' tilt restricts diaphragmatic movement, compromises respiration and may restrict venous return.
- Tracheal intubation and ventilation are usually used.
- Nitrous oxide is avoided.
- Complications include: absorption of CO_2, accidental subcutaneous or extra-peritoneal insufflation, local trauma with the trocars and scopes, and covert bleeding.
- Postoperative pain management includes local infiltration of the scope insertion points, NSAIDs, paracetamol and sometimes morphine infusions.
- Monitor temperature, as some children become pyrexial during the prolonged surgery.

Repair of inguinal hernia, orchidopexy, hydrocele repair

These are common procedures with similar anaesthetic requirements. Surgery is via a small lower abdominal incision and most are day cases in otherwise healthy children.

Neonatal hernias are very common, especially in premature babies. These are not day case procedures. Inguinal hernias in infants and children are usually painless and easily reducible on the ward. If a hernia is irreducible, strangulation of bowel may occur, and surgery becomes more urgent.

Orchidopexy is required if the testis is high in the scrotum or intra-abdominal, as late malignant change is a risk in the undescended testis.

Anaesthetic considerations

- Inhalational or IV induction.
- Airway management with a face mask or LMA™.
- Small babies may require tracheal intubation and ventilation.
- Pre-emptive analgesia with NSAIDs and paracetamol is useful, either on ward or after induction of anaesthesia.
- Analgesia is with local anaesthetic, either ilioinguinal nerve block, local infiltration or caudal block.
- For a bilateral surgery, a caudal block may be preferable as it is easily achieved and has a predictable effect.
- Bradycardia can occur with peritoneal traction during surgery for orchidopexy.
- During orchidopexy the scrotal skin may not be adequately anaesthetized with an ilioinguinal block and additional local infiltration of the scrotal incision is useful.
- Occasionally, the testis is high, or intra-abdominal, in which case repair is done as a two-stage procedure. Initially, the testis is brought to the inguinal ring and at a later date it is brought into the scrotum.
- Laparoscopic repair in all age groups is becoming more popular; the additional considerations for this type of surgery are listed above.

Torsion of the testis

This can occur in the neonate but mostly in young children. Repair is a surgical emergency or the testis may be damaged permanently.

Anaesthetic considerations

- Assume the child has delayed gastric emptying.
- Use a rapid sequence, or modified rapid sequence, induction.
- Intubate the trachea; control ventilation.
- Analgesia as for orchidopexy.

8

Anaesthesia for specific neonatal conditions

Inguinal hernia repair

Inguinal hernia is particularly common in the premature neonate (5% if < 1500 g). The incidence is increased with decreasing age, in the small-for-dates neonate and in males. Abdominal contents are frequently in the sac, but are not usually obstructed, and can be reduced with analgesia and local pressure on the sac. Repair is usually done electively. Occasionally, there is incarceration of the bowel which may result in strangulation of the bowel as the blood supply is compromised. Emergency surgery is indicated and bowel resection may be necessary

Anaesthetic considerations

Most centres use general anaesthesia but some advocate spinal anaesthesia.

General anaesthesia involves:

- Either a gaseous or IV induction.
- Intubation and ventilation.
- Opiates are not required.
- Local anaesthetic blocks. These may include caudal, ilioinguinal or local infiltration.
- Postoperative analgesia is with paracetamol and occasionally codeine.

Spinal anesthesia has been used extensively in some centres. However, surgery may be prolonged and the duration of the spinal can be insufficient. Protagonists believe it is safer because it is associated with fewer perioperative apnoeas and episodes of bradycardia than general anaesthesia. This advantage is lost if any sedative medication is used.

Pyloric stenosis

This condition affects 1 in 250 babies (see Box 8.1). It is most common in boys, especially the first-born male. Presentation is usually in the first few weeks of life as hypertrophy of the muscle layer in the pylorus increases. Features include vomiting, classically projectile, weight loss and later dehydration.

Due to persistent vomiting the child may also develop:

- hypokalaemia
- metabolic alkalosis
- hypochloraemia.

It may be possible to palpate the pyloric mass during a test feed and peristaltic movements may be seen in the abdomen. Ultrasound is commonly used to identify the mass and barium contrast studies are usually unnecessary. Emergency surgery is not indicated. It is important to correct the metabolic abnormalities before surgery, which may take 1–3 days. IV fluid regimens vary, but essentially water, sodium and potassium need to be replenished and renal function will adjust the acid–base status gradually. Five per cent dextrose in 0.45% saline, with added potassium, is used as the main IV fluid. In addition, measured gastric losses are replaced with 0.9% saline.

Surgery is not considered until:

- serum Cl^- > 89 mmol/l
- no residual acidosis
- serum potassium is within the normal range
- serum bicarbonate < 30 mmol/l.

In the past, pyloromyotomy was done using local anaesthetic infiltration. More recently, mini-laparotomy has become standard but the procedure can also be done laparoscopically.

Anaesthetic considerations
Preoperative
- Optimize fluid, electrolyte and acid–base status.
- Regular aspiration of the nasogastric tube, in addition to free drainage of gastric contents.
- Stomach washouts.

Perioperative
- Aspirate the nasogastric tube (NGT) and preoxygenate.
- Induction and maintenance vary widely. Generally, a rapid sequence induction is performed (thiopentone, suxamethonium, cricoid pressure) thought atracurium is also frequently used. A gaseous induction is sometimes appropriate.
- Opiates are not usually required.
- Blood loss is minimal.
- Extubate awake, in lateral position.
- Infitration of local anaesthetic into wound provides adequate analgesia.

Postoperative
- Leave NGT to drain.
- Use paracetamol.
- Continue IV fluids until able to feed.
- Apnoea is common, possibly related to cerebrospinal fluid electrolyte shifts.

Box 8.1   Incidence of congenital abnormalities

Congenital abnormality	Incidence
Pyloric stenosis	1 : 250
Tracheo-oesophageal fistula and oesophageal atresia	1 : 3000
Diaphragmatic hernia	1 : 4000

Tracheo-oesophageal fistula (TOF) and oesophageal atresia (OA)

There are five main types of TOF, by far the commonest being oesophageal atresia with a distal TOF – 85% of cases.

Forty per cent of babies have an associated congenital anomaly, particularly malrotation of the gut, duodenal abnormalities, imperforate anus or cardiac disease. The VATER association is a well-recognized condition:

- **V**ertebral abnormalities usually hemivertebrae
- **A**nal atresia
- **T**racheo-oesophageal fistula
- **R**adial hypoplasia/renal dysplasia.

Antenatal diagnosis of TOF due to polyhydramnios, or detection of associated abnormalities on ultrasound, is often possible.

Clinical features of TOF, or OA, depend on the type of fistula but may include:

- Choking with the first feed.
- Respiratory distress at birth due to excess secretions, which cannot be swallowed, with coughing, choking, vomiting and/or cyanosis.
- Abdominal distension.
- Babies with the H-type fistula may present late with persistent cough and recurrent chest infection.
- X-ray changes – a nasogastric tube is noted coiled up in the blind upper pouch. In type 2 (OA without a fistula) there is no stomach air bubble on X-ray. Rarely, dye is needed to identify the anatomy.

Mortality is uncommon. Survival is related to the size of the baby and to the presence of associated abnormalities, which must be sought. A cardiac echocardiogram should be done, as 35% of babies with TOF or OA have congenital cardiac abnormalities. There is an increased incidence of prematurity, or affected babies may be small for their gestational age.

Following diagnosis, a Replogal (multiple-ended suction catheter) is placed and suction applied to keep the upper pouch clear. Babies are nursed head up to decrease the risk of aspiration. Surgical closure of the fistula, via a right thoracotomy, is required, preferably with anastamosis of the two ends of the oesophagus. The gap between the proximal and distal oesophagus may be too great and the proximal end is either ligated or brought out in the neck as a stoma. A gastrostomy is undertaken, pending definitive surgery later.

Anaesthesia considerations

Main problems are:

- Prematurity and associated concerns such as bronchopulmonary dysplasia, the effects of repeated aspiration.
- Associated conditions such as renal or cardiac abnormalities.
- Practical difficulties related to airway management. There is a risk of intubating the fistula, which will make ventilation impossible. There is also a risk, even if the tracheal tube is placed correctly, that anaesthetic gases will enter the stomach causing distension and impairing ventilation.
- Many surgeons do a bronchoscopy or oesophagoscopy to try to identify the fistula before repair.

Preoperative

- If intubation is required before surgery, care must be taken to avoid gastric distension either by accidentally intubating the fistula or using high pressures via the face mask.
- Use atropine premedication.
- IV access.
- Ensure blood is available.

Perioperative

- Inhalational induction and maintenance of spontaneous respiration. Avoid manual ventilation as this may distend the stomach and make ventilation difficult.
- Awake intubation is now rarely used.
- Paralysis with suxamethonium or atracurium and intubation. Classically, the bevel of the tracheal tube is placed posteriorly to avoid intubating the fistula.
- Oxygen, air and isoflurane are used. Nitrous oxide is avoided.
- Manual ventilation is often used, so compliance changes can be rapidly identified. Also, during surgery, the lung is compressed to achieve adequate surgical access. Occasionally, ventilation is not adequate and surgery stops whilst conditions are adjusted to achieve efficient ventilation. Once the fistula is occluded, ventilation is more stable.
- An arterial cannula is useful.
- If the baby is to be woken up after surgery, small doses of fentanyl 1–3 µg/kg are used perioperatively. Lumbar or caudal epidural catheters have been used successfully and may decrease the incidence and duration of postoperative ventilation. Alternatively, local infiltration of the wound is used with a morphine infusion post operatively (see below).
- If the baby is to remain ventilated postoperatively, fentanyl 10–20 µg/kg can be used.

Postoperative

- Approximately 50% of babies return to the intensive care unit and remain ventilated. This is either because of their size and general condition, or because the anastamosis is considered tight and muscle relaxation and ventilation are continued for several days.
- If not ventilated, morphine infusions (nurse-controlled analgesia) are used and babies cared for in a high-dependency unit.
- Paracetamol.

Late complications

- Oesophageal strictures are common and repeated oesophageal dilatations are necessary.
- Many children retain a persistent cough ('TOF cough'). Some may continue to aspirate because of altered oesophageal motility and poor reflexes.

Diaphragmatic hernia (DH)

This occurs when there is herniation of the abdominal contents through the diaphragm. It is most commonly left-sided as 70% of DH occur through the posteriorly placed foramen of Bochdalek. Associated abnormalities occur in 50% of patients and include neural tube defects, malrotation of the gut, cardiac and renal abnormalities. Most babies present at birth with cyanosis and respiratory distress. The condition occurs early in development of the foetus and the affected lung is hypoplastic.

The degree of respiratory compromise is related to the extent of this hypoplasia. In addition, pulmonary hypertension (PHT) persists in the neonatal period and acute pulmonary hypertensive crisis can occur. Other clinical features include: scaphoid abdomen, decreased breath sounds on the affected side, displaced heart sounds and, rarely, bowel sounds in the chest.

Most affected babies require ventilation at birth but occasionally babies with small defects present later with difficulties in feeding and increasing respiratory distress. Outcome, and the extent of respiratory support required to maintain adequate gas exchange, are related to the severity of pulmonary hypoplasia. Conventional ventilation, high-frequency ventilation, oscillation or rarely extracorporeal membrane oxygenation (ECMO) may be indicated. Babies who require ECMO often have a poor outcome.

Surgery to close the DH is deferred until the baby is stable and can maintain reasonable blood gases on moderate levels of respiratory support and without severe PHT crises. Surgical repair is by laparotomy.

Anaesthesia

- Transfer to theatre intubated, paralysed and sedated.
- Nasogastric tube on free drainage.
- Laparotomy in the supine position.
- Cross-match blood.
- Air/oxygen/isoflurane; avoid nitrous oxide which could increase gut distension.

- Fentanyl 10–25 µg/kg.
- Good venous access and an arterial cannula.
- There is an increased risk of pneumothorax.
- Most patients require extended ventilatory support postoperatively, sometimes many weeks.

Abdominal wall defects: gastroschisis, exomphalos

The aetiology of these two conditions differs (see Box 8.2) but the anaesthetic management is similar:

Box 8.2   Abdominal wall defects; gastroschisis, exomphalos

Defect	Incidence	Associated features
Gastroschisis Gut herniation via abdominal wall defect	1 : 5–10 000	No covering sac Prematurity 60% Intestinal atresia or stenosis in 15%
Exomphalos (omphalocele) Gut herniates via the umbilical cord	1 : 6000	Gut contained within a sac of peritoneum and amniotic membrane, which may have ruptured. Prematurity 10% Gastrointestinal defects in 30% Congenital heart disease in 20% Beckwith–Wiedemann syndrome in 10%

- The defect in the abdominal wall must be closed soon after birth. With large defects, there is a rapid loss of fluid and resuscitation with albumin may be required. The exposed tissue is covered with moist swabs or occlusive dressing to decrease these losses.
- Electrolyte imbalance can occur and should be corrected preoperatively.
- Cross-match blood.
- Monitor blood glucose regularly.
- Place a nasogastric tube and aspirate.
- Associated conditions should be determined.

Sometimes the defect can be closed at the first operation. Some babies with small defects can breathe spontaneously after surgery but the majority require ventilation. This is due to increased intra-abdominal pressure when the gut is returned to the abdomen, with compromised lung function. A subgroup of babies have large defects and primary closure is impossible. They have a synthetic mesh silo bag placed around the edges of the defect and the bag is slowly wound down, gently pushing the gut back into the abdomen over many days, until eventually closure of the skin edges is possible.

Anaesthesia

In addition to the usual requirements of the neonate:

- Babies are usually ventilated postoperatively.
- Anaesthesia involves muscle relaxation, isoflurane in air and oxygen.
- Avoid nitrous oxide which could increase gut distension.
- Use fentanyl 10–20 µg/kg.
- Careful replacement of blood and fluids.
- IV access placed in the upper limbs is ideal as abdominal pressure may restrict venous return temporarily immediately after surgery.
- Arterial cannula is necessary.
- Epidurals have been used successfully in a few centres, especially if extubation is likely within the first 2 postoperative days.
- Postoperative morphine infusions are commonly used.
- If longer-term ventilation is necessary, morphine infusion and sedation are required.

Later closure of the abdomen when a silo has been used involves the same management and blood loss can be significant.

Laparotomy

Indications for laparotomy in the neonate include intestinal stenoses or atresia, malrotation, duplication cysts, colostomy and necrotizing enterocolitis (see Box 8.3).

Preoperatively, the babies are assessed for:

- prematurity
- coagulopathy
- volume status
- sepsis
- associated congenital abnormalities.

Box 8.3   Intestinal abnormalities requiring laparotomy in neonates

Condition	Associated conditions	Special features
Intestinal atresia, jejunal, ileal	• Atresia or stenosis may occur, can be multiple	• Antenatal polyhydramnios • Distended abdomen with intestinal obstruction
Duodenal atresia	• Premature babies • Down's syndrome • Other gut abnormalities, imperforate anus	• Antenatal polyhydramnios • Bile-stained vomit
Malrotation, volvulus	• Associated with diaphragmatic hernia, other gut abnormalities	• Abdominal distension, dilated bowel on X-ray • Vomiting • Perforation – peritonitis
Meconium ileus	• Cystic fibrosis	

Anaesthesia

- Ensure blood is available.
- Risk of aspiration; place a NGT tube, rapid sequence induction (RSI) (or modified RSI).
- If sepsis is present, avoid central neuroaxial blocks due to risk of thrombocytopaenia and coagulopathy.
- If the baby is to be extubated at the end of surgery, take care with opiate dose.
- Use small doses of opiates if sepsis is present.
- Many require postoperative ventilation.
- Epidurals often useful if no contraindications.

Necrotizing enterocolitis

This condition commonly affects premature or low birth weight babies. It can result in gut perforation, peritonitis and septic shock. There is an increased incidence following birth asphyxia or hypotensive episodes.

Babies are often very sick with sepsis, poor cardiac output, coagulopathy and thrombocytopenia. Abdominal X-ray reveals air in the gut wall or free gas in the abdomen. Surgery is necessary if there are areas of ischaemic gut (see Laparotomy above). Resuscitation requires blood products and volume expansion. Epidural is contraindicated.

Colostomy

Colostomy is required for various conditions including Hirschprung's disease (aganglionic segment of bowel), which results in intestinal obstruction, abdominal distension and failure to pass meconium. Colostomy is performed early and the abnormal segment of gut is resected later. Anaesthetic requirements are as for laparotomy. Blood loss can be sufficient to require transfusion.

Rectal biopsy, anorectal malformation such as imperforate anal membrane

Minor procedures such as these are brief and are usually done using a face mask or a laryngeal mask. If the site of surgery is appropriate, a caudal or spinal can be used as the sole anaesthetic.

9

ENT, dental and cleft palates

These procedures are very common in young children. Many are treated as day cases. The main issue is good access to the airway for the surgeon whilst maintaining anaesthesia and protecting the airway from blood and debris during surgery.

Adenotonsillectomy (T&A)

Some centres treat selected patients for adenoids or T&A as day cases, particularly in North America. Most children in the UK stay overnight. A small group of patients have important co-morbid disease.

Recurrent infection is the main indication for surgery. Children < 3 years having tonsillectomy usually have obstructive symptoms.

Occasionally children have marked upper airway obstruction and obstructive sleep apnoea (OSA).

Obstructive sleep apnoea

Features:

- Snoring.
- Interrupted sleep, which may result in behavioural problems.
- Periods of apnoea, resolving spontaneously.
- Intermittent hypoxia.
- Sleep studies reveal the frequency and duration of apnoea and the associated decrease in oxygen saturation.
- In severe OSA, chronic hypoxia can result in pulmonary hypertension, cor pulmonale and right heart strain (identified on electrocardiogram (ECG)).
- Children may fail to thrive and develop facial abnormalities.
- Sedative premedication should be avoided and opiates used with great care.
- Obstructive symptoms do not resolve immediately postoperatively. If the child is small, < 3 years, they may need to be monitored in a high-dependency unit/paediatric intensive care unit (PICU) postoperatively because of the risk of airway problems.

Anaesthesia for adenotonsillectomy

- Premedication can be used, providing there is no OSA.
- IV or gaseous induction.
- LMA™ used in some centres.
- Alternatively, intubation with an RAE-pattern tube, fixed at the centre of the lip for placement of the mouth gag.
- Spontaneous respiration or intermittent positive-pressure ventilation (IPPV) with muscle relaxants.
- Opiate (codeine or fentanyl), paracetamol and non-steroidal anti-inflammatory drugs started at the beginning of the operation provide effective pain relief into the postoperative period.
- Postoperative nausea and vomiting (PONV) common (increased after fentanyl).
- Give IV fluids.
- Give dexamethazone as antiemetic.

Postoperative bleeding may be:

- *Early*, within the first 4–6 h, due to primary haemorrhage (< 1% of operations).
- *Late*, secondary haemorrhage due to infection over following 1–2 weeks.

Features include:

- bleeding, may be concealed and the actual amount underestimated
- pallor, decreased capillary refill
- tachycardia
- hypotension
- nausea
- vomit of blood.

Management

- Establish monitoring of blood pressure, heart rate.
- Insert IV cannula, give fluids to correct hypovolaemia before surgery.
- Check haemoglobin and cross-match blood.
- Check clotting.
- Assume the child has a full stomach with swallowed blood.
- Check emergency equipment, suction.
- There are two main schools of thought about the induction of anaesthesia:

1. Rapid sequence induction with preoxygenation, cricoid pressure, IV induction and intubation following suxamethonium.
2. Gas induction with sevoflurane or halothane, cricoid pressure, direct laryngoscopy and, if the larynx is visible, give suxamethonium and intubate the trachea.

Many advise using the left lateral, slightly 'head-down' position for induction and intubation. However, if the anaesthetist is inexperienced in intubation in this position, it is safer to use the more familiar supine position.

In addition:

- Blood may be required.
- Use a large orogastric tube to help remove blood from the stomach.
- If adenoidal bleeding does not stop, nasopharyngeal packs are occasionally required. These are left for 24 h to provide local pressure to the adenoidal bed.

Ear surgery
Minor ear surgery
This includes placement of grommets, T tubes, simple repair of the tympanic membrane and examination of ears. These are short procedures usually undertaken as day cases:

- premedication usually not required
- IV or gas induction is appropriate
- anaesthesia by face mask or LMA™
- simple analgesics
- rapid recovery.

Major ear surgery
Mastoidectomy, myringoplasty, otoplasty (repair of bat ears), ear reconstruction:

- surgery may be prolonged
- premedication useful
- balanced technique with inhalational agent and opioids
- nitrous oxide is avoided if the middle ear is entered
- 'head-up' position
- avoid hypertensive episodes
- mild hypotension, e.g. labetolol
- antiemetic, high incidence of PONV

- IV fluids
- analgesia includes local infiltration or nerve block, paracetamol, diclofenac, opiates.

Nasal cautery

Nose bleeds are frequent in children and occasionally require cautery to Little's area of the nasal septum. This is done as an elective procedure, and a throat pack is used.

Choanal atresia

Unilateral or bilateral. Often associated with syndromes, e.g. CHARGE. Babies nose breathe, so if bilateral atresia is present, acute airway obstruction occurs. This requires placement of an oral airway and early surgery. Surgery involves drilling out the choanal tract.

Anaesthetic considerations

- Oral tracheal tube (e.g. RAE-pattern or flexometallic).
- Throat pack.
- After surgery, nasal stents are left in place.
- Recurrent dilatations may be required.

Microlaryngoscopy and bronchoscopy

A mainly diagnostic procedure to identify airway pathology, bronchoscopy is described below. To examine the larynx, the tracheal tube may need to be completely withdrawn into the pharynx. If spontaneous respiration is maintained via the tube, and effective analgesic of the larynx with lignocaine is achieved, the procedure is well tolerated.

If laser treatment is planned for airway papilloma, granuloma or cysts, a metallic laser tube is used. The child's face is protected with saline swabs and the eyes with saline swabs or eye shields. One hundred per cent oxygen is avoided because of the risk of airway fires.

Infections, epiglottitis and croup

Epiglottitis

- Caused by haemophilus influenzae.
- HiB vaccine is protective.
- Peak incidence 3–6 years.
- Child looks unwell, is miserable with fever, drooling and stridor.
- Risk of acute complete airway obstruction, so **DO NOT**:

- insert an IV cannula
- send the child for an X-ray
- examine the throat.

Management
- avoid stress
- gas induction with sevoflurane or halothane
- continous positive airways pressure (CPAP)
- avoid muscle relaxants
- continue spontaneous respiration
- intubate with deep inhalational anaesthesia (typically there is a large, red, swollen epiglottis visible during direct laryngoscopy)
- antibiotics
- sedation and supportive therapy in PICU
- ensure accidental extubation does not occur
- IPPV usually not necessary
- rapid recovery.

Croup (laryngotracheobronchitis)
- usually viral, parainfluenzae
- rarely diptheria-protective effect of vaccination
- peak incidence 2–4 years
- mild systemic disturbance
- fever, cough.

Management
- croup is common and about 1% will require admission
- humidified oxygen
- intubation
- sedation and supportive therapy
- steroids
- slow recovery.

Foreign bodies (FB)
- a common paediatric accident
- FB can be aspirated or swallowed
- peak incidence 9–24 months
- 50% FB are foods, e.g. nuts or sweets
- 50% environmental, e.g. toys, pen tops, stones
- may be asymptomatic, so diagnosis is delayed

- features include wheeze, cough, stridor
- can cause complete obstruction leading to hypoxia and respiratory arrest.

X-ray changes include:

- FB may be seen
- area of collapse/consolidation
- hyperinflation on the affected side if the FB prevents full expiration
- Mediastinal shift

Management
If in extremis, use resuscitation guidelines, choking algorhithm.
Chest X-ray in inspiration and expiration (unilateral hyperinflation).
Atropine premedication.
Monitored gas induction

Then:

Bronchoscopy for FB in the airway
- Topical lignocaine to larynx.
- Initial placement of a tracheal tube.
- Withdraw tube and surgeon inserts the bronchoscope.
- Spontaneous respiration via bronchoscope, assisted when necessary.
- Jet ventilation can be dangerous in children because of risk of pressure damage (pneumothorax, pneumomediastinum, potential obstructed expiration), so usually avoided.
- Removal of FB may be a long procedure.
- Re-intubate at the end of procedure or allow to wake up using a face mask.
- Treat stridor if present.

Oesophagoscopy for FB in the digestive tract
- Ensure you can ventilate the lungs.
- Use a muscle relaxant.
- Intubate the trachea.
- Place tracheal tube to the side of the mouth to allow good access for the oesophagoscope.

Complications
Accidental extubation perioperatively.
Oesophageal perforation – mediastinitis, pneumomediastinum.

The difficult paediatric airway

Most children who have difficult airways, or who will be difficult to intubate, are predictable, as they fit into one of the following groups:

1. Facial abnormalities (usually related to syndromes) resulting in:
   - mandibular hypoplasia
   - microsomia.
2. Restricted mouth opening:
   - temperomandibular joint fusion
   - burns.
3. Restricted neck movement:
   - known neck instability, e.g. Down's syndrome
   - fusion, e.g. postcervical surgery, juvenile rheumatoid arthritis, bony neck abnormalities.
4. Soft tissue swelling:
   - mucopolysaccharidoses
   - cystic hygroma
   - haemangioma
   - subglottic stenosis.

Most children, even if difficult to intubate, do not have airways that are difficult to manage.

Assessment

History:

- Documented difficulties from previous anaesthetic.
- Previous postoperative problems, e.g. PICU admission, oxygen therapy.
- Syndrome or condition known to be associated with airway difficulties.
- Previous long-term intubation or neonatal intubation (risk of acquired subglottic stenosis).
- Respiratory pattern/respiratory distress.
- Stridor.
- Sleep apnoea.
- Oxygen dependence.

Examination

Tests used in adult practice for evaluating the difficult airway have not been validated for paediatric practice. It is useful, however, to check the degree of mouth opening, the visibility of palatal structures (Mallampatti) and neck movement.

Management

- Ensure adequate help and necessary equipment is available.
- Have a clear plan for anaesthesia; discuss fully with team.
- Premedication with atropine, oral or IM.
- Inhalational induction with sevoflurane or halothane.
- Assess the airway when asleep – can the child's chest be readily ventilated by hand? If not, decide whether the next step is to wake the child up?, do a tracheostomy?
- Does the child need tracheal intubation?
- Would an LMA™, face mask or nasal prong be suitable for airway management?
- Consider using suxamethonium and tracheal intubation.
- Otherwise, deepen the anaesthetic and do a direct laryngoscopy.
- Intubation aids include:
  - bougie
  - alternative laryngoscopes, (straight blade, curved blade, McCoy, Bullard)
  - fibreoptic scopes.

Paediatric fibreoptics

Useful for:

- tracheal intubation
- diagnostic:
  - airway abnormalities – dynamic or structural
  - infection, bronchial lavage, diagnostic sampling
  - foreign bodies
  - during surgery – to review the airway during complex surgery for tracheomalacia.

Diagnostic fibreoscopy can be done in the sedated child but for intubation anaesthesia is usually necessary (see Box 9.1). A method of maintaining the airway, ensuring adequate oxygenation and continuing anaesthesia must be found. This can be by face mask, nasal prong or LMA™ using sevoflurane, halothane or isoflurane in oxygen.

Stridor

Stridor is defined as noisy breathing associated with obstructed airflow. It can be inspiratory, expiratory or mixed. The aetiology is different in the neonate and child (see Box 9.2).

Anaesthesia for a child with stridor:

- Atropine premedication (for the vagolytic effect and to dry the mucous membrane so that topical lignocaine is effective).
- Avoid sedation.
- Gaseous induction.
- Maintain spontaneous respiration until diagnosis is clear.

Box 9.1   Paediatric scopes

	2.2 mm FOS	3.8 mm FOS
Advantages	Flexible in small infants and children Can take tracheal tube 2.5 mm	More robust Better optics as more fibreoptic bundles Has side channel – useful for suction, insufflation of O_2, diagnostic lavage, instillation of local anaesthetic ('spray as you go') Channel can be used to take a wire as aid to intubation
Disadvantages	Difficult to manoeuvre No suction channel	Too large for small children Takes tracheal tubes above 4.5 mm if required.

Box 9.2   Stridor in the neonate and child

Neonate	Infant and child
Laryngomalacia Tracheomalacia Subglottic stenosis (congenital or acquired following tracheal intubation) Subglottic haemangioma Congenital cysts Vascular ring	Infection, e.g. croup, epiglottitis, diphtheria, bacterial tracheitis, local abscess, laryngeal papilloma Trauma, e.g. foreign body, neck trauma, following intubation – postextubation stridor Tumour Angioedema

Postintubation/extubation stridor

Common especially in younger patients. Management includes:

- Oxygen.
- Humidification.
- CPAP.
- Nebulized epinephrine 5 ml of 1 in 1000 adrenaline (epinephrine) with 5 ml saline, (monitor ECG during nebulizer, stop if heart rate > 180 bpm or dysrhythmias occur).
- Dexamethasone.

Tracheostomy

Used for:

- Inadequate upper airway, e.g. severe retrognathia or micrognathia, Pierre–Robin, Treacher–Collins.
- Chronic lung disease, long-term ventilation required.
- Subglottic stenosis.
- Vocal cord palsy.
- Laryngomalacia.
- Obstructed airway, e.g. papilloma.
- To facilitate major head and neck surgery, e.g. craniofacial reconstruction.

A paediatric tracheostomy is performed at the level of the second to third tracheal ring. There are many different tracheal tube designs and sizes.

Anaesthesia for tracheostomy

Rarely possible to perform awake in children.

Ideally, the trachea is intubated for a tracheostomy, but if this is difficult or even impossible, it is reasonable to manage the airway during surgery with any of the following:

- face mask
- nasal prong airway
- LMA™.

Local infiltration is used for postoperative analgesia. Spontaneous respiration or IPPV is used depending on circumstances. Usually, anaesthetic agent in oxygen +/− air, but avoid nitrous oxide and give 100% O_2 when changing to the tracheostomy tube. Ensure lungs are ventilated and clear, and that capnography trace is present after insertion of tracheostomy tube.

Complications

There is morbidity and mortality associated with tracheostomy, including:

- Haemorrhage.
- Infection.
- Pneumothorax (check chest X-ray after the procedure).
- Accidental displacement of tracheostomy tube, either completely dislodged or displaced into a false track subcutaneously.
- Tube obstruction with airway secretions (ensure use of humidified gases).
- Granuloma at tracheostomy stoma.
- Tracheal stenosis.
- Death <1% per year.

Dental procedures

Most paediatric dental work is done in the awake child using local anaesthetic. Recent guidelines have formalized procedures so that all dental anaesthetics must be undertaken in hospitals with suitable paediatric provision. Following public concern at the deaths of several children during dental anaesthesia (five children died between 1996–1999), the report 'A Conscious Decision' recommended that:

1. General anaesthesia should be used for dental treatment only when clinically necessary. The alternative is local anaesthesia or conscious sedation.
2. Other methods of pain and anxiety management should be used whenever possible.
3. All general anaesthesia for dental surgery should be done in a hospital.
4. In common with all other specialist areas of anaesthesia, anaesthetists should be trained for dental anaesthesia, equipment must be maintained and skilled assistance should be available.

Anaesthesia may be required for extraction of carious or broken teeth, orthodontic extractions, exploration of cysts or complex fillings. General anaesthetics are also required in children who cannot cooperate with awake dental procedures either because of their age, physiological or psychological compromise or learning difficulties.

The main issues to consider are:

- Shared access to the mouth/airway.
- Risk of aspiration of blood, debris or loose teeth – always use a throat pack.
- Pain – simple analgesics usually sufficient, local anaesthetic blocks are placed by the surgeon. Fentanyl is used in more extensive procedures.
- PONV.

Most patients are treated as day cases and the general principles for provision of anaesthesia to this group apply.

Simple extractions of first teeth can be managed with an LMA™, intermittent mask or nasal prong anaesthesia. Use of a nasal tracheal tube is convenient if extensive dental procedures are planned in several quadrants of the mouth. Alternatively, if the nasal route is contraindicated (e.g. known coagulopathy, small nasal passages, previous pharyngoplasty), an RAE-pattern tube fixed at the corner of the mouth is usually satisfactory.

Cleft lip and palate

Incidence 1:500 babies, varying severity, occasionally airway management or intubation may be difficult. 20% have an associated syndrome e.g. Pierre Robin. Anaesthetic Management:

Cleft lip is repaired in first three months:

- Atropine premedication.
- Inhalational induction.
- Oral RAE tube and throat pack.
- Spontaneous or assisted ventilation.
- Analgesia with fentanyl, paracetamol and LA (infiltration or infraorbital bock).
- Postoperatively – paracetamol and codeine.

Palate repair at about nine months:

- Anaesthesia as above but some repairs are extensive.
- Group and save or cross match – may need blood.
- Analgesia: fentanyl, LA, paracetamol.
- Post operatively – morphine infusion or codeine, plus paracetamol.
- IV fluids per operatively but can drink soon post operatively.
- Extubate awake.

10

Anaesthesia for urology

Children presenting for surgery on the renal tract account for a large part of the paediatric anaesthetist's workload. Procedures undertaken range from minor surgery in well children, such as cystoscopy or circumcision, to major surgery in children who may have renal failure.

Minor procedures
- cystoscopy
- resection of posterior urethral valves
- circumcision
- insertion of suprapubic catheter
- hypospadias repair
- orchidopexy.

In general, these children are well and require routine preoperative evaluation. Sedative premedication and/or local anaesthetic cream for IV induction is applied as indicated.

Cystoscopy
Indications for cystoscopy are very varied from minor haematuria or difficulty in passing urine to follow-up after reconstructive or tumour surgery.

Anaesthesia
- Spontaneous respiration with a laryngeal mask airway or face mask.
- Cystoscopy may produce a marked physiological response resulting in hyperventilation and tachycardia.
- Morphine 20–30 μg/kg IV is sometimes useful to improve intraoperative conditions and postoperative pain relief. It should be given several minutes before the start of the procedure as it has a relatively slow onset. Alternatively, codeine phosphate can be used.
- Prophylactic antibiotics are often required to prevent a Gram-negative bacteraemia.

Resection of posterior urethral valves (PUV)

An abnormal flap of tissue is present in the urethra of male neonates and leads to obstruction to urine flow. The resulting back-pressure in the renal tracts can lead to bilateral hydronephrosis and renal damage. PUV may be diagnosed in the antenatal period but is more commonly diagnosed in the neonate or young infant. The earlier the diagnosis is made and obstruction relieved by resection of the valves the better, the chances of good recovery of renal function. Late diagnosis may result in chronic renal failure.

Anaesthesia
- Resection of PUV is a cystoscopic procedure.
- Preoperative assessment of renal function.
- In very small infants (< 5 kg) tracheal intubation is undertaken. Larger infants can be managed with an LMA™ and spontaneous ventilation.
- Caudal analgesia provides excellent pain relief.
- Antibiotics are given.
- Careful postoperative fluid management is required if large volumes of urine are produced after relief of the obstruction.

Hypospadias repair

Hypospadias occurs when the external urethral opening is proximal to the urethral tip. Hypospadias refers to a spectrum of conditions from the very mild through to the severe. It is not commonly associated with other major systemic disease. A number of different operations are undertaken to repair the defect. Occasionally, additional tissue is required to repair larger defects and graft tissue may be taken from the buccal mucosa. Minor hypospadias can be managed on a day-stay basis. Renal function is not impaired.

Anaesthesia
- Usually with LMA™ and spontaneous ventilation.
- Caudal analgesia provides excellent analgesia and the addition of clonidine extends its duration.
- If buccal mucosa is used, intubation is required with controlled ventilation. Nasal intubation is most convenient for the surgeon, but oral intubation with an RAE tube positioned to one side of the mouth is also acceptable. A throat pack is advisable as there may be bleeding into the mouth. Local anaesthetic with adrenaline (epinephrine) is injected to reduce bleeding and provide postoperative analgesia.

- Simple analgesics paracetamol and diclofenac provide additional analgesia.
- Prophylactic antibiotics are given.

Orchidopexy

This operation is performed for undescended testis. Surgery usually involves an inguinal incision and a small scrotal incision. The testis is located in the inguinal canal and brought down and secured in the scrotum. If the testis is intra-abdominal, laparoscopy is used to occasionally check the postion and a two-stage operation is used. In the first stage, a transverse low abdominal incision is required and the testis is located and moved to the inguinal region. In the second stage, done some time later, the testis is moved to the scrotum (the two-stage Fowler–Stephens operation).

Anaesthesia

- Simple orchidopexy is performed with spontaneous ventilation with an LMA™.
- In unilateral surgery an ilioinguinal local anaesthetic block is commonly used. This does not block pain from the small scrotal incision but in practice this is unimportant. For bilateral orchidopexy a caudal block is more common.
- For first-stage Fowler-Stephens or laparoscopy, tracheal intubation and controlled ventilation is required.

Major urological procedures

- pyeloplasty
- nephrectomy or heminephrectomy
- ureteric reimplantation
- closure of bladder extrophy
- bladder augmentation and formation of a Mitrofanoff channel
- excision of Wilm's tumour (nephroblastoma)
- genitoplasty
- renal transplantation.

Pyeloplasty, nephrectomy and heminephrectomy

Pyeloplasty is performed to relieve obstruction of the flow of urine at the pelviureteric junction. The abnormality is usually unilateral and does not compromise renal function. Until recently, most pyeloplasties were open procedures with the patient positioned almost lateral over a small bolster. More recently, some are done laparoscopically.

A nephrectomy or heminephrectomy is performed either for hydronephrosis or to remove a non-functioning kidney or the part of the kidney which is non-functioning. An increasing number of these operations are also undertaken laparoscopically.

Anaesthesia
- Tracheal intubation with controlled ventilation.
- Bleeding is seldom a problem with pyeloplasty or nephrectomy but is more common with heminephrectomy.

The following is a guide to cross-matching blood:

- Pyeloplasty: no cross-match.
- Nephrectomy: group and save.
- Heminephrectomy: cross-match required.
- There is debate about the best form of postoperative analgesia for open procedures. Some anaesthetists advocate an opiate-based technique, others use an epidural-based technique. Either technique is effective.
- If the procedure is undertaken laparoscopically, field blocks or local infiltration can be used followed by simple analgesics in combination with either morphine infusion (patient-/nurse-controled analgesia, PCA/NCA) or codeine.

Ureteric reimplantation

Ureteric reimplantation is performed to abolish uretovesical obstruction which may be unilateral or bilateral. Renal function may be compromised and should be checked preoperatively. Reimplantation takes place either as an isolated procedure or part of a major reconstruction and usually involves a lower abdominal transverse incision with the patient supine.

Anaesthesia
- Tracheal intubation with controlled ventilation.
- Bleeding is seldom significant.
- Postoperative pain is ideally managed with a continuous epidural, but morphine infusion, PCA or NCA is also effective.

Bladder extrophy

This rare congenital abnormality affects between 1 in 20 000 and 1 in 50 000 live births and boys three times more commonly than girls. The bladder is laid open on the anterior abdominal wall. There is complete epispadias and the pubic bones are widely splayed making surgical closure difficult. If closure is delayed more than 48 h, the condition of the bladder deteriorates, it becomes progressively more hyperaemic and oedematous, and the risk of infection increases. Delayed closure also increases the risk of renal damage because of obstruction to urine flow in the urethra and of bladder carcinoma in later years.

The diagnosis is commonly made in the antenatal period by ultrasound scan.

Preoperatively, the defect is covered with a thin plastic film to prevent fluid and heat loss and to reduce the risk of infection. Renal function is checked and blood cross-matched.

The surgical approach to bladder extrophy is still evolving and varies. The aim of surgery is to close the bladder, appose the pelvic bones, repair the epispadias and produce continence with a bladder of adequate volume. The surgical debate centres largely on the timing and extent of surgery. Some surgeons advocate radical surgery in the neonatal period while others adopt a more limited approach with simple bladder closure and more radical surgery postponed to 6 months or a year.

Simple bladder closure is relatively quick ($\pm$ 2 h) and not associated with large blood or fluid losses. At the end of surgery, a plaster of paris hip spica is applied. These children often require surgery later in life mainly for bladder augmentation and attempts to achieve continence.

Anaesthesia
The surgery intended determines the anaesthetic approach.

For simple bladder closure:

- All the considerations of neonatal anaesthesia apply.
- Tracheal intubation and controlled ventilation.
- Good IV access (avoid the femoral vessels because of proximity to surgical field).
- Careful temperature control.
- Epidural analgesia with plain bupivacaine.
- Cross-match 1 unit of blood, but bleeding usually not extensive.
- Postoperative ventilation seldom required.

For radical surgery (bladder closure, epispadias repair, pelvic osteotomies), all the considerations for simple bladder closure, but in addition:

- Arterial cannula and central venous catheter (avoid femoral vessels).
- Expect large blood losses.
- Postoperative ventilation common.
- As postoperative ventilation is likely, an opiate-based technique is appropriate (fentanyl or morphine).

Wilm's tumour (nephroblastoma)

Wilm's tumours (nephroblastoma) account for more than 50% of abdominal tumours in children. They usually occur in children < 5 years of age and may be bilateral in 5–10% of cases. These tumours commonly present with a palpable abdominal mass, but can also present with fever, abdominal pain or haematuria. Hypertension may occur as a result of renal ischaemia, mediated by the renin–angiotensin system.

Wilm's tumour may be associated with:

- aniridia (congenital absence of the iris)
- hemihypertrophy
- Beckwith–Wiedeman syndrome
- neurofibromatosis
- acquired von Willibrand's disease.

Treatment depends on the histology and staging of the tumour but is often with chemotherapy followed by surgical excision and radiotherapy. Preoperative chemotherapy usually reduces the size and vascularity of the tumour.

Anaesthesia
- Children may recently have completed chemotherapy and careful review of the blood count and clotting is required.
- If chemotherapy has been undertaken, a Hickman line will be in situ and can be used for induction of anaesthesia and monitoring of central venous pressure (CVP). If no Hickman line is present, a central line should be inserted.
- Hypertension is likely and this should be reviewed with the antihypertensive therapy. Control of blood pressure intra-operatively is occasionally required.
- Blood should be cross-matched and major bleeding anticipated; massive bleeding is unusual.
- Direct arterial access for pressure monitoring and blood sampling is required.

- Urinary catheter.
- Good IV access in upper limbs (it may be necessary to clamp the inferior vena cava (IVC)).
- A large transverse abdominal incision is used.
- Epidural analgesia provides excellent intra- and postoperative analgesia.
- Intraoperative cardiovascular instability can arise from compression of the IVC.
- Postoperative ventilation is seldom required.

Intersex and genitoplasty

The topic of intersex is complex, full of controversy, and beyond the scope of this book. For the children and families, there are difficult psychological problems and decisions. There are a number of causes of ambiguous genitalia, the most common of which is congenital adrenal hyperplasia (CAH or adrenogenital syndrome). CAH results from a deficiency of 21-hydroxylase, which results in low levels of cortisol. This causes the pituitary to secrete large amounts of adrenocorticotropic hormone (ACTH) stimulating the production of large quantities of androgenic steroids. These children may present as neonates with a salt losing crisis. Female infants become virilized with clitoral hypertrophy and/or labial fusion and it is these girls that require a feminizing genitoplasty. Children with CAH are treated with corticosteroids to reduce ACTH production and may also need mineralocorticoids.

Anaesthesia

- Steroid cover is needed if steroids are taken. The endocrine team advise on steroid cover and fluid management in the perioperative period.
- The difficult psychological aspects of this type of surgery must be recognized.
- Tracheal intubation with controlled ventilation; surgery is extensive and long.
- Bleeding makes surgery more difficult and moderate induced hypotension can be helpful. This is usually combined with infiltration of local anaesthesia with adrenaline (epinephrine) to reduce bleeding.
- Continuous epidural or caudal analgesia provides excellent intraoperative conditions and postoperative pain control.

Renal failure

Causes of chronic renal failure in children:

Acquired glomerular disease:
- glomerulonephritis
- glomerulosclerosis.

Developmental renal disease:
- pyelonephritis secondary to reflux and/or infection
- posterior urethral valves
- hereditary renal disease
- nephropathies
- polycystic renal disease.

Miscellaneous:
- haemolytic uraemic syndrome
- vascular nephropathies.

Systemic effects of chronic renal failure (CRF)

Anaemia – normal haemoglobin concentration in these patients is 6–7 g/dl.
This is due to:

- reduced erythropoietin production
- reduced red cell survival
- iron and folate defeciency.

Coagulopathies are due to:

- platelet dysfunction
- increased capillary fragility
- thrombocytopenia secondary to bone marrow depression.

Fluid and electrolytes abnormalities:

- fluid overload
- hyperkalaemia
- hypocalcaemia with risk of osteoporosis
- hyperphosphataemia
- hypo- or hypernatraemia depending on renal disease.

Acid/base abnormalities:

- metabolic acidosis
- low plasma bicarbonate.

Cardiovascular abnormalities:

- cardiac failure
- hypertension; may be severe and difficult to control
- risk of dysrhythmias
- pulmonary congestion.

Growth and development:

- stunted growth
- delayed development.

Neurological:

- peripheral neuropathy
- encephalopthy
- siezures.

Reduced immunity.

Renal transplantation

Renal transplantation accounts for the majority of solid organ transplantation in children. As expertise has improved, and with the introduction of effective immunosuppression, graft survival is now about 95% at 1 year and 85% at 5 years.

Anaesthetic management
Preoperative
- Preoperative review of the patient concentrates on the effects of chronic renal failure.
- Determine the fluid and electrolytes and acid–base status of the child. Pretransplant dialysis may be required. The condition of the patient should be discussed with the renal team.
- Determine the site of any vascular shunt and avoid IV or arterial cannulae close to this site.
- Ensure familiarity with the institution's transplant protocol.

Intraoperative
- Induction and maintenance of anaesthesia should maintain cardiovascular stability.

- Invasive monitoring with arterial cannula and CVP catheter is required, avoid shunt or potential shunt sites.
- Epidural analgesia is generally avoided because of the use of heparin and the risk of coagulopathy associated with CRF.
- CVP is maintained at 10–12 cmH$_2$O to optimize renal perfusion.
- Transfuse red cells to haematocrit of 35–40% according to local protocols.
- Before release of cross-clamp, most protocols use frusemide 1 mg/kg, mannitol 1 g/kg and dopamine at 5 µg/kg/min.
- Release of the vascular clamps often results in hypotension as the new kidney fills with blood. In addition, the fluid used to preserve the transplanted kidney is potassium rich and can cause dysrhythmias. Ensure adequate filling before clamp release; give blood and fluid aggressively, if necessary.
- The problems of reperfusion of the grafted kidney are more severe in small children receiving large kidneys.

Postoperative
- Postoperative ventilation is sometimes necessary if large kidneys have been placed in small children or if aggressive fluid management has led to pulmonary oedema.
- Careful attention to fluid management.
- Good postoperative analgesia with morphine infusions, PCA or NCA, is required.

11

Anaesthesia for paediatric cardiac surgery

Anaesthesia for paediatric cardiac surgery: general considerations

Preoperative preparation

The aims of the preoperative visit include:

- Assessing and understanding the pathophysiology and general physical condition of the patient.
- Prescribing premedication and giving other preoperative instructions.
- Giving information and answering questions.
- Building rapport with child and family.
- Formulating an anaesthetic plan.

Information about the child's condition is gathered from the notes. In particular, echocardiographic and catheter data should be reviewed as well as other investigations including the chest X-ray and electrocardiogram (ECG). A history and examination should be performed.

Particularly assess:

- cardiac failure
- cyanosis
- current medication
- potential veins (prescribe EMLA or ametop to specific vein).

Premedication

Premedication (see Box 11.1) is probably unnecessary in infants < 4 weeks but is not contraindicated. Premedication should be omitted, or used sparingly, in children in severe cardiac failure. Local anaesthetic cream is useful in all children even if a gaseous induction is planned because it allows insertion of the IV cannula at a much lighter plane of anaesthesia. Sedative premedication may be particularly beneficial in patients whose cyanosis is worsened with crying, e.g. tetralogy of Fallot. Older children may be very anxious and also benefit from premedication.

Box 11.1   Suggested premedication for cardiac surgery

Age	Weight (kg)	Drug	Dose (mg/kg)	Comments
< 4 weeks		No premed		EMLA or ametop only
From 4 weeks to 6 kg		Triclofos	50–75	
	6–15	Triclofos	50–75	
	> 15	Midazolam	0.5–1.0	Max 15 mg
		Temazepam	0.5–1.0	Max 20 mg

Induction

Intravenous ketamine produces rapid hypnosis and good analgesia without respiratory or cardiovascular depression. It should be avoided in patients with severe valve stenosis as the tachycardia and increased myocardial oxygen consumption are detrimental. Thiopentone and propofol are widely used, but cause a dose-dependent decrease in blood pressure and must be used with caution in children with impaired cardiac function. Other agents commonly used include fentanyl, midazolam and etomidate. Careful titration of all IV drugs is essential.

Sevoflurane is the volatile agent of choice for gaseous induction but after intubation isoflurane is often used in low concentrations. Isoflurane and sevoflurane are well-tolerated at low inspired concentrations. Intubation may be oral or nasal. Positive-pressure ventilation with an appropriate concentration of oxygen in air is used. Nitrous oxide is usually avoided because of the risk of air bubbles entering the circulation during cardiac surgery.

A non-depolarizing muscle relaxant is used for intubation. Vecuronium or pancuronium are both suitable. Pancuronium is longer lasting and causes a tachycardia, but this is well-tolerated by children. Pancuronium in combination with fentanyl produces very stable cardiovascular conditions with little change in heart rate or blood pressure.

Monitoring

Routine monitoring should start before induction of anaesthesia wherever possible.

In addition to routine monitors the following are used:

- Central venous pressure (CVP) (internal jugular, subclavian, femoral, umbilical venous catheter)
- direct arterial pressure (radial, femoral, axillary, umbilical arterial catheter)
- temperature (nasopharyngeal, skin)
- urinary catheter
- transoesophageal echo (used increasingly in paediatric practice).

Management of cardiac bypass (CPB) in children

- Anaesthesia is maintained with fentanyl 10–50 µg/kg which may be combined with midazolam 50–100 µg/kg and low concentrations of isoflurane 0.2–0.75%. In addition, when on CPB, isoflurane is added to the pump in a concentration of 0.5–1.0%.
- Blood loss is usually minimal pre-CPB. Careful monitoring is required while dissection around the great vessels occurs and during aortic and venous cannulation. The cannulae may obstruct venous return or left ventricular outflow causing a fall in cardiac output.

Aprotinin is used in most redo operations and in small infants having major surgery. It reduces postoperative bleeding and decreases the systemic inflammatory response to CPB.

Before bypass:

- The activated clotting time (ACT) and baseline arterial gases should be checked.
- Give heparin 3 mg/kg.
- Aim for an ACT of 400 sec or at least three times the baseline.
- Give additional fentanyl, midazolam and muscle relaxant just before bypass.
- Give antibiotics according to local protocol.

Institution of bypass:

- Hypotension secondary to acute haemodilution may occur.
- Vasoconstrictors (phenylephrine 1–5 µg/kg, metaraminol 1–10 µg/kg) may be required to maintain perfusion pressures.
- Hypotension may be secondary to collateral flow to the lungs. All shunts should be ligated by the surgeons before CPB.
- Ventilation is discontinued during bypass.
- If the surgery requires the heart to be stopped, myocardial protection is achieved by aortic cross-clamping with infusion of cardioplegia

into the coronaries via the aortic root. Blood cardioplegia is given from the pump by the perfusionist, but crystalloid cardioplegia may be given by the anaesthetist.

During bypass:

- Monitor ACT and acid–base status.
- Monitor perfusion pressure. Perfusion pressures vary depending on the age of the patient. Lower pressures are used in neonates compared with older children. Vasoconstrictors (see above) or vasodilators glyceryl trinitrate 1–10 µg/kg/min or phentolamine 10 µg/kg may be required.
- The temperature varies with the complexity of the repair. Most surgery is performed at 25–32°C although deep hypothermia to 16–18°C is used for circulatory arrest.
- Potassium ± magnesium, calcium and sodium bicarbonate are given as required

During rewarming and before weaning from bypass:

- Ensure blood and blood products are available.
- Inotropes and vasodilators ready to infuse.
- Ventilate the lungs and suction the endotracheal tube.
- Ensure normal acid–base and electrolytes.
- Core temperature 36°C and core/peripheral difference < 4°C.

Post bypass:

- The heart is filled by restricting the venous drainage from the heart to the pump.
- After weaning from CPB pump, blood is transfused via the aortic cannula to ensure adequate filling as measured by CVP, right atrium (RA) or left atrium (LA) pressure.
- Modified ultrafiltration (MUF), may be used (see below).
- When MUF is complete, protamine 3–6 mg/kg is given slowly via a peripheral vein.
- It is very important that the perfusionist and surgeons are aware that protamine is being given so that pump suckers can be turned off. This is to ensure that no protamine reaches the pump circuit in case it is necessary to go back on CPB.
- Check ACT and blood gases.

- Blood products, red cells and colloid are given as indicated.
- The thromboelastogragh is useful in guiding the use of blood products post-CPB.

Coagulation disorders are more common with:

- Prolonged bypass.
- Infants < 8 kg.
- Cyanotic patients.

Transfer to intensive care unit (ICU):

- Monitoring is transferred to a portable monitor.
- Blood or colloid should be available during transfer.
- Emergency drugs available.
- Manual ventilation.
- ICU should be aware of arrival; ventilator and equipment prepared.
- Rapid transfer of monitoring in ICU.
- Comprehensive handover to nurse and intensivist.

Cardiopulmonary bypass

The principles of CPB in children are similar to those in adults but there are special considerations. These include the need for small prime volumes to reduce the effects of haemodilution, the use of higher flow rates, the use of deep hypothermic cardiac arrest and the use of modified ultrafiltration post-CPB.

Hypothermia protects the brain and other important organs from ischemic damage during CPB. Moderate hypothermia is defined as a core temperatures of 25–30°C, while profound hypothermia is 15–20°C. Deep hypothermic cardiac arrest at 15°C provides a bloodless field but is now rarely used.

Hypothermia in conjunction with the non-pulsatile flow of bypass impairs flow in the microcirculation, which can lead to areas of hypoperfusion with sludging. The optimal haematocrit post-CPB in children has not been determined but, if the child remains cyanotic, a high haematocrit is desirable, 45–50%, whereas a much lower haematocrit is accepted in patients without cyanosis and with good myocardial function.

CPB prime

In adults, the priming volume represents about 30% of the blood volume. In neonates or infants, the priming volume can exceed the blood volume by 200–300%. This results in substantial haemodilution with thrombocytopenia, hypoproteinaemia, a reduction in clotting factors and anaemia, which all contribute to the coagulopathy associated with CPB.

In small infants, blood is almost always added to the prime and colloid may also be used. Mannitol is sometimes included to promote a diuresis.

Modified ultrafiltration (MUF)

After CPB in children, there is an excess of total body water and the haematocrit is low. MUF removes excess body water to increase the haematocrit. Blood is taken from the patient through the arterial cannula after CPB. This blood is then passed through an ultrafilter where filtrate is removed and the haemoconcentrated blood returned to the patient via the right atrium.

There are benefits from ultrafiltration including:

haemodynamic
- ↑ Blood pressure
- ↑ CO
- ↓ pulmonary vascular reistance (PVR)
- ↓ heart rate

metabolic
- ↓ total body water

haematalogical
- ↑ haematocrit
- ↓ transfusion requirement.

MUF may be associated with a shorter period of postoperative ventilation and decreased ICU stay. It has not been shown to reduce mortality.

Classification of congenital heart disease

Classification of Congenital Heart Disease:

1) 'Simple' left-to-right shunt: increased pulmonary blood flow:
   - arial septal defect (ASD)
   - ventricular septal defect (VSD)
   - patent ductus arteriosus (PDA)
   - endocardial cushion defect, e.g. atrioventricular septal defect (AVSD)
   - aortopulmonary window (AP window).

2) 'Simple' right-to-left shunt: decreased pulmonary blood flow with cyanosis:
   - tetralogy of Fallot (TOF)
   - pulmonary atresia
   - tricuspid atresia
   - Ebstein's anomaly.
3) Complex shunts: mixing of pulmonary and systemic blood flow with cyanosis:
   - transposition of great arteries
   - truncus arteriosus
   - total anomalous pulmonary venous drainage
   - double-outlet right ventricle
   - hypoplastic left heart syndrome.
4) Obstructive lesions:
   - aortic stenosis
   - mitral stenosis
   - pulmonary stenosis
   - coarctation of aorta
   - interrupted aortic arch.

Management of specific lesions

1) 'Simple' left-to-right shunt
Clinical features may include
- high pulmonary blood flow
- heart is volume loaded
- cardiac failure resulting in:
  - breathlessness
  - difficulty in feeding
  - failure to thrive
  - recurrent chest infection
  - hepatomegaly
  - cardiomegaly
  - pulmonary plethora
- murmur.

Risk of pulmonary hypertension can lead to reversal of intracardiac shunt to become (R → L) – Eisenmenger's syndrome. The onset of Eisenmenger's syndrome implies severe pulmonary hypertension which usually means the cardiac lesions is inoperable, the only alternative is heart–lung transplantation.

Management of children with L → R shunts includes diuretics, with or without digoxin, to treat the cardiac failure. In some cases, surgical palliation is undertaken before definitive surgery. This involves the application of a pulmonary artery band which reduces the diameter of the pulmonary artery and thus pulmonary flow, which in turn reduces the shunt and prevents the development of pulmonary vascular disease. The child has time to grow without the development of pulmonary hypertension until definitive surgery is undertaken.

Atrial septal defect (ASD)
Most ASDs are now closed percutaneosuly in the catheter laboratory. Occasionally, surgery is required for larger defects.

Ventricular septal defect (VSD)
Four types of VSD are described, depending on their position: supracristal, infracristal (80%), canal type and muscular. The size of the VSD determines the size of the shunt and thus the clinical features. Large VSDs are termed non-restrictive and small VSDs called restrictive.
    Large non-restrictive lesions often result in preoperative heart failure and these patients are at risk of postoperative pulmonary hypertension. Some small VSDs will close spontaneously.

Atrioventricular canal defect (AVSD)
AVSD may be complete, with an ASD, VSD and cleft mitral valve, or partial with a primum ASD and cleft mitral valve. AVSD is commonly associated with Down's syndrome and with a relatively large shunt. Surgery is usually planned around 3–6 months of age before the onset of pulmonary vascular disease.

Patent ductus arteriosus (PDA)
A PDA is essential for the fetal circulation but usually closes soon after birth. Failure of the PDA to close results in a left-to-right shunt with increased pulmonary blood flow and possible heart failure. Indomethacin is used to promote closure in neonates. If this fails, surgery is required, which is performed through a thoracotomy. PDAs are common in small premature babies and may also be present in older children, when they are usually closed percutaneously by a cardiologist.

Anaesthetic considerations
• Omit or reduce premedication in patients with severe heart failure.

- IV induction may be slow because of dilution through the pulmonary circulation.
- Accidental injection of air may result in it crossing to the systemic circulation and entering the coronary or cerebral circulation causing ischaemia.
- Antibiotics for endocarditis prophylaxis.
- Careful induction of anaesthesia for those in severe failure. Limit the concentration of volatile anaesthetic agent used. The severity of right ventricular failure is sometimes underestimated.
- Opiates help to maintain cardiovascular stability.

Particular postoperative problems following repair of left-to-right shunts
- Pulmonary hypertension. This may be treated by:
  - high inspired oxygen concentration
  - low PCO_2
  - correct acidosis
  - deepen sedation or anaesthesia. Fentanyl is particularly useful.
  - Vasodilators, e.g. milrinone
  - Nitric oxide.
  - Arrhythmias, particularly supraventricular tachycardia (SVT), and atrioventricular conduction abnormalities, are common following surgery near the conduction system of the heart. Most arrhythmias are temporary but occasionally complete heart block occurs and permanent pacing is required.
- Atrioventicular valve incompetence after repair of AVSD.

2) 'Simple' right-to-left shunts
The predominant feature of these conditions is hypoxaemia with cyanosis. This results from a shunting of blood from the right to left side of the heart and also a reduction in the pulmonary blood flow.

In these conditions in the neonatal period, pulmonary blood supply may be dependent on flow through a PDA. If so, an infusion of prostaglandin E1 is started to maintain ductal patency before surgery to establish a palliative systemic → pulmonary artery shunt (Blalock–Taussig shunt). This shunt increases pulmonary blood flow and improves oxygenation. Definitive repair is carried out later when the child is bigger.

Tetralogy of Fallot (TOF)
The four features of the tetralogy are:

- VSD
- overriding aorta
- right ventricular outflow tract obstruction (RVOTO)
- right ventricular hypertrophy.

'Spelling' in tetralogy

The RVOTO may be due to valvular, supravalvar or infundibular stenosis. The infundibular stenosis is usually dynamic and constriction will cause a hypercyanotic episoder or 'tet spell' by reducing pulmonary blood flow and increasing R $\rightarrow$ L shunt. Precipitating factors include high PCO_2, low pH and surgical stimulation. Older children with tetralogy will tend to squat during a spell. This increases the systemic vascular resistance by reducing blood flow to the legs. The increased SVR reduces the R $\rightarrow$ L shunt, increasing the pulmonary blood flow and improving cyanosis.

Usually definitive surgery is carried out in the neonatal period. If this is not possible, a systemic $\rightarrow$ pulmonary artery shunt is done first, with definitive surgery postponed until the child is bigger.

Management of hypercyanotic spells during anaesthesia:

- 100% oxygen
- hyperventilation
- IV fluid (10 ml/kg bolus)
- fentanyl for sedation
- consider sodium bicarbonate
- vasoconstriction to $\uparrow$ systemic vascular resistance (SVR), thus $\downarrow$ R $\rightarrow$ L shunt
  - noradrenaline 0.5 µg/kg bolus then 0.1–0.5 µg/kg/min
  - phenylephrine 5 µg/kg bolus then 1–5 µg/kg/min
- beta blockers; relax infundibular spasm and $\downarrow$ heart rate
  - propanolol 0.1–0.3 mg/kg bolus

Following successful repair of tetralogy of Fallot, 'spelling' does not occur.

Anaesthetic considerations in right-to-left shunts

- Premedication is helpful in promoting a smooth induction to minimize cyanosis.
- Avoid air bubbles in venous cannulae which may cross to cerebral and coronary circulations.
- Endocarditis prophylaxis is essential.
- Gas induction is slower because of reduced pulmonary blood flow.

- IV induction is more rapid.
- High inspired oxygen concentrations and low $PaCO_2$ reduce the PVR and increase blood flow to the lungs by reducing $R \rightarrow L$ shunt.

3)   Complex shunts
Transposition of the great arteries
This is the most common cause of neonatal cyanotic CHD. The aorta originates from the right ventricle and the pulmonary artery comes from the left ventricle. Two parallel circuits are present and mixing must occur to allow survival. There is often a VSD present, but in the absence of a VSD mixing can occur through a PDA or ASD. If mixing is inadequate, an emergency balloon atrial septostomy is done in the neonatal period to enlarge the intra-atrial communication. TGA is corrected by the 'arterial switch' operation when the aorta and pulmonary arteries are disconnected from their incorrect ventricles and reattached to their correct ventricles. The most important and difficult part of this operation is the reattachment of the coronary arteries.

Hypoplastic left heart syndrome
In this condition the left ventricle is severely hypoplasic, as are the proximal aorta, aortic valve and the mitral valve. The neonate depends for its survival on mixed blood from the right ventricle and pulmonary artery flowing through the large PDA into the distal aorta (duct-dependent circulation). The degree of mixing depends on the size of the ASD. All these babies die without surgery, usually within the first month of life. The surgical options are heart transplantation or a Norwood procedure. The Norwood procedure has three stages and results ultimately in a Fontan circulation.

4)   Obstructive lesions
Obstruction to the outflow from a ventricle increases the load on the ventricle and if severe results in ventricular failure. The most important lesions are left sided.

Coarctation of the aorta
Three types of coarctation exist:

- preductal (infantile type)
- postductal
- juxtaductal.

Preductal (infantile) coarctation
This is associated in 90% of cases with other lesions such as VSD or PDA. A tight coarctation results in cardiac failure and blood flow to the lower body is through the PDA, which in neonates is kept patent with an infusion of prostaglandin E1 (PGE1). Severe cases warrant preoperative ventilation and inotropes to support cardiac function until surgery is performed. Cardiovascular collapse will occur if the duct closes.

Anaesthetic considerations
- These patients are often very sick.
- Surgery is performed through a left thoracotomy.
- During surgery, lung retraction takes place and ventilation may be compromised. It is important that the endotracheal tube does not have a large leak.
- The arterial cannula and pulse oximeter are on the right arm (preductal). All other pulses will disappear while clamping the aorta during the repair.
- Allow patient to cool – 34°C before clamping of aorta to reduce risk of ischemic damage to spinal cord.
- On release of the clamp, anticipate hypotension ± bleeding. Give fluids before clamp release.
- Cardiovascular instability may follow surgery and inotropes or vasodilators may be required.
- Postoperative ventilation is usually required.

Postductal and juxtaductal coaratation (adult type)
These patients are most frequently diagnosed because of upper limb hypertension and present much later.

Aortic stenosis
There are three types of congenital aortic stenosis:

- valvular (80%)
- subvalvular
- supravalvular.

Neonates with critical aortic stenosis are in cardiac failure and can be very sick. Older children are often asymptomatic but may have episodes of syncope or angina and are at risk of sudden death.

Anaesthetic considerations

- Avoid vasodilation, negative inotropy, tachycardia and bradycardia as coronary perfusion may be compromised.
- Opiate-based induction and anaesthesia.
- Maintain PGE1 in neonates before surgery.
- Postoperative hypertension in older children may be a problem.
- Patients with William's syndrome also have coronary anomalies, and sudden cardiac arrest has been reported associated with anaesthesia.

Common surgical procedures in paediatric cardiac surgery

Modified Blalock–Taussig shunt (BT shunt) :

Connecting the subclavian artery to the pulmonary artery using a small gortex graft creates this systemic-pulmonary shunt. It is almost always performed in the neonatal period or in early infancy, to provide a pulmonary blood supply in cyanotic infants. It is used as temporary palliation to allow the child to grow before a more definitive repair is carried out. It can be used, for example, on a child with pulmonary atresia, tricuspid atresia or tetralogy of Fallot.

Glenn shunt

The Glenn shunt is the first stage of the Fontan circulation (see below). The SVC is connected to the right pulmonary artery (RPA) to provide a blood supply to the RPA. SVC blood flow to the lungs is now passive, nonpulsatile, at systemic venous pressure and is only possible if PVR is low. In small children, flow in the SVC is greater than in the IVC, so a substantial pulmonary blood flow is achieved.

Fontan circulation or Total cavo-pulmonary connection (TCPC)

The Fontan circulation (TCPC) is the next stage after a Glenn shunt and results in a functional univentricular heart. The SVC is already connected to the pulmonary artery (Glenn) and the Fontan is the connection of the IVC to the pulmonary artery. This results in all the systemic venous blood being directed to the pulmonary arteries. It is important to appreciate that whatever the original cardiac lesion, the Fontan operation results in a functional single ventricle. The single ventricle is used to pump blood to the systemic circulation, and blood flow to the lungs is passive from the SVC and IVC.

Cardiac catheterization

Transthoracic echocardiography is very useful in investigating cardiac disease but cardiac catheterization is necessary to obtain more detailed information about the cardiac status of a patient. The heart is most commonly accessed via the femoral artery and vein. In older cooperative children, this can be achieved by local anaesthesia alone, but in younger children general anaesthesia or sedation is required. These children may be very ill preoperatively, in cardiac failure, or profoundly cyanosed, or have poor ventricular function. In addition, the catheter itself may cause deterioration in cardiovascular function, particularly if arrhythmias occur. The injected contrast is hypertonic and may induce cardiac instability or a large diuresis. Heparin 1 mg/kg is used if the femoral artery is entered. Antibiotics are usually not given.

Anaesthetic Considerations
- Aim for stable haemodynamic conditions.
- Inspired oxygen concentration close to 21%.
- Positive-pressure ventilation with tracheal intubation is the most widely used technique but in some patients a spontaneously breathing technique with an LMA^{TM} can be used.
- PCO_2 similar to preanaesthetic conditions.
- The use of opiates is probably unnecessary as catheterization is not a painful procedure. Paracetamol and local anaesthetic infiltration are usually adequate pain relief postoperatively.

Interventional cardiac catheterization
Interventional cardiology is an expanding field. An increasing number of complex procedures are undertaken in the catheter laboratory.
    Examples include:

- occlusion of PDA
- closure of ASD and VSD
- ballooning of valves, e.g. aortic and pulmonary valves
- Balloon ± stenting of recoarctation or conduit.

During cardiac catheterization, sudden deterioration can occur as a result of arrhythmia, rupture and bleeding, or obstruction of flow. It may occasionally be necessary to institute bypass in an emergency. These patients may be very ill with poor ventricular function or critical valve stenosis. A transoesophageal echo (TOE) is often used to guide the

Box 11.2   Dental surgery

Patient category	>10 yrs	5–10 yrs	<5 yrs
A Not allergic to penicillin and penicillin not more than once in the previous month If at special risk use **B** or **C** If allergic to penicillin use **C**	Ampicillin 1 g IV at induction and Amoxycillin 500 mg PO 6 h later **OR** Amoxycillin 3 g oral 4 h preop and same dose as soon as possible post op	Ampicillin 500 mg IV at induction and Amoxycillin 250 mg PO 6 h later **OR** Amoxycillin 1.5 g oral 4 h preop and same dose ASAP postop	Ampicillin 250 mg IV at induction and Amoxycillin 125 mg PO 6 h later **OR** Amoxycillin 750 mg oral 4 h preop and same dose ASAP postop
Special risk patients* **B** Not allergic to penicillin and penicillin not more than once in previous month	Ampicillin 1 g IV at induction and Gentamycin 2 mg/kg IV then Amoxycillin 500 mg PO 6 h later	Ampicillin 500 mg IV at induction and Gentamycin 2 mg/kg then Amoxycillin 250 mg PO 6 h later	Ampicillin 250 mg IV at induction and Gentamycin 2 mg/kg IV then Amoxycillin 125 mg PO 6 h later
C Allergic to penicillin or penicillin more than once in past month	Teicoplanin 400 mg IV at induction and Gentamycin 2 mg/kg IV **Single dose only**	Teicoplanin (< 40 kg) 10 mg/kg IV at induction and Gentamycin 2 mg/kg IV **Single dose only**	Teicoplanin 10 mg/kg IV at induction and Gentamycin 2 mg/kg IV **Single dose only**

*Patients with intracardiac prosthetic material and/or previous endocarditis are at special risk.

placement of interventional devices and, if the child is small, the TOE probe can occlude or displace the tracheal tube. Blood should be available if bleeding is a possibility. All resuscitation drugs and a defibrillator must be present. The anaesthetic management of these patients depends on the underlying pathology. Heparin is given if the femoral artery is entered and antibiotics are given to reduce the risk of endocarditis.

Patients having cardiac catheters, for diagnostic or interventional reasons, should be closely monitored in the postoperative period for:

- bleeding from arterial and venous puncture sites
- blood pressure and pulse
- ECG and pulse oximetry
- foot pulses and leg perfusion (arterial spasm or thrombosis).

Other procedures which may occur in the catheter lab include:

- Electrophysiological studies and ablation of aberrant pathways in patients with arrhythmias. These are often long procedures and patients should be intubated and ventilated.
- Cardioversion. May be an emergency so patient may have a full stomach. If not, a single dose of propofol and 100% oxygen will suffice.
- Pericardiocentesis. These patients may have a low cardiac output and care with induction is needed.

Antibiotic prophylaxis for procedures under general anaesthesia

Dental surgery – see Box 11.2
Other surgery

- Gastrointestinal surgery: Use **B** or **C** as above depending on penicillin allergy and exposure.
- Genitourinary surgery/instrumentation: use **B** or **C** as above depending on penicillin allergy and exposure.
- Surgery/instrumentation of upper respiratory tract: As for dental surgery.

12

Anaesthesia for paediatric neurosurgery

Intracranial pressure (ICP) and cerebral blood flow in children

The contents of the cranium consist of:

- brain tissue 80%
- blood 10%
- CSF 10%.

Raised ICP results form an increase in any of these three components.

Cerebral blood flow (CBF)

Cerebral blood volume is determined by CBF. CBF is regulated by the metabolic demands of the brain ($CMRO_2$), intracerebral acidosis and $PaCO_2$. It is also subject to autoregulation which allows CBF to remain relatively constant across a wide range of arterial pressures.

- CBF is higher in children (approx 100 ml/100 g/min) than in adults (approx 60 ml/100 g/min).
- Autoregulation occurs at a lower mean arterial pressure in children compared with adults, as low as 40 mmHg in small children.
- In premature neonates, autoregulation does not occur and CBF is proportional to arterial pressure.
- Intracerebral steal may occur with vasodilation of normally reactive blood vessels. This reduces flow in vessels that have lost the ability to autoregulate, for example vessels to tumours or those affected by trauma and infection.
- Inverse cerebral steal occurs when normal blood vessels constrict, resulting in preferential flow to abnormal vessels.

Intracranial pressure

In older children and adults the cranium has a fixed volume. An increase in the volume of the blood, cerebrospinal fluid (CSF) or brian tissue will lead to an increase in ICP.

- In young children the suture lines are not yet fused and an increase in intracranial volume in possible without a corresponding increase in ICP.
- The normal ICP in neonates is 2–4 mm Hg (± 15 mmHg in adults).

Cerebrospinal fluid

The CSF, is produced continuously by the choroid plexus at a rate sufficient to exchange the volume five times a day. Production of CSF in children is affected by age and pathophysiology but is not affected by changes in intracranial pressure. CSF production can be temporarily reduced by drugs such as frusemide, steroids and acetazolamide. CSF is reabsorbed by the arachnoid villi at a relatively fixed rate that may be reduced by intracranial infection, haemorrhage or malformation, all of which are more common in children.

Hydrocephalus may be caused by reduced absorption, increased production or obstruction to flow of CSF.

Clinical features of raised ICP

Clinical features of raised ICP include:

- vomiting
- irritability or drowsiness
- bulging fontanelle and eyes
- increasing head circumference
- downward gaze of eyes (setting sun sign)
- ↑ blood pressure, ↓ heart rate (Cushing's response) usually occur late.

Anaesthetic management for craniotomy

The most common indication for craniotomy in children is tumour; other indications include epilepsy, head injury, vascular lesions and craniosynostosis.

Tumour

Malignancy is second only to accidents as a cause of death in children. Tumours in the central nervous system are the most common form of malignancy after leukaemia. About 60% of intracranial tumours occur in the posterior fossa with the peak incidence between the ages of 1 and 8 years.

Preoperative assessment and premedication

In addition to the standard preoperative assessment the neurosurgical patient requires an assessment of their neurological state:

- Changes in conscious level.
- Evidence of raised ICP.
- Presence of focal neurology such as cranial nerve palsies or bulbar palsies. Bulbar palsies may have led to aspiration and lung damage, particularly in smaller children.

Some neurological conditions are associated with other pathologies:

- Small expremature babies requiring ventriculo-peritoneal shunt surgery as a result of intraventicular haemorrhage and hydrocephalus frequently have bronchopulmonary dysplasia. They may be on long-term oxygen and require postoperative ventilation.
- A cerebral abscess may be secondary to congenital heart disease or associated with sickle cell disease.
- Renal infection and damage may be present in patients with spinal cord abnormalities.
- Latex allergy is more common in patients with spina bifida and those with myelomenigocele

In patients with raised ICP, sedative premedication is avoided as this may further increase the ICP and slow recovery from anaesthesic.

If ICP is normal, sedative premedication can be used. LA creams are used in all children even if an inhalational induction is planned. Their use enables cannulation to take place at a much lighter plane of anaesthesia. Atropine and other antisialogogues are now seldom used.

Induction

Induction of anaesthesia can be intravenous or inhalational. It is important to minimize increases in ICP during induction of anaesthesia. A calm inhalational induction is preferable to the relentless pursuit of IV cannulation in a screaming child!

The increase in blood pressure associated with laryngoscopy and intubation can be attenuated with a short-acting opioid such as fentanyl or alfentanil and by ensuring an adequate depth of anaesthesia. Lignocaine 1.5 mg/kg given IV 3 min before intubation is also effective.

A reinforced armoured tracheal tube is used for neurosurgery to avoid kinking during surgery. It must be securely fastened to ensure that it is not displaced. The securing tapes should be waterproofed so that secretions or other fluids do not loosen them during surgery when access to the head is limited.

Any of the newer non-depolarizing relaxants can be used. Suxamethonium is rarely used for routine cases.

Maintenance

A balanced anaesthetic is often used with a combination of an opioid, such as fentanyl, and low concentrations (<1 MAC) of volatile agents, such as isoflurane or sevoflurane, with muscle relaxation and controlled ventilation. If there is a high risk of air embolism, nitrous oxide should not be used.

Total intravenous anaesthesia with propofol and a short-acting opioid, such as remifentanil, may be used, especially in older, larger patients.

Surgery on the brain tissue is relatively non-stimulating and light planes of anaesthesia are sufficient. There are several periods during surgery that are very stimulating. These include:

- Insertion of the pins from the cranial frame, to position the head.
- During skin incision. Stimulation can be reduced by infiltration of local anaesthetic.
- During opening of the dura mater.
- During wound closure.

At these times, a bolus of opioid may be required.

Generally, normocapnia is maintained with hyperventilation reserved for acute increases in ICP, or if the ICP is very high. Good communication with the surgeon is essential. Many anaesthetists allow the core temperature to drift towards 35°C in the belief that this will afford some cerebral protection.

The use of frusemide, mannitol, steroids and antibiotics during craniotomy depends on local guidelines.

Profound induced hypotension is rarely used in paediatric neuroanaesthesia but hypertension due to inadequate anaesthesia must be avoided. Hypertension may result from direct stimulation of cardiovascular centres in the brain stem even with adequate anaesthesia, and the surgeon must be informed of these changes.

Monitoring

In addition to routine monitoring, the following may be required in major neurosurgical cases:

- Arterial cannula.
- Urinary catheter for long cases or where high urine outputs are anticipated.
- Central venous catheter if large blood losses are expected. A femoral catheter may be preferable to one in the internal jugular vein as venous drainage from the head may be reduced. If a central venous pressure (CVP) catheter is inserted to aspirate air, it must be accurately placed in the right atrium with X-ray control.
- Precordial Doppler is used in some centres for the detection of air emboli. However, it is an extremely sensitive monitor and its clinical usefulness debatable.

Fluid balance

- Fluid requirements during paediatric neurosurgery are generally small.
- Overtransfusion of fluid should be avoided as this may lead to increased brain oedema. 0.9% sodium chloride solution is the fluid of choice.
- Glucose containing fluids should not be used as hyperglycaemia is associated with a worse neurological outcome after brain injury.
- Hyper- or hypo-osmolar fluids should not be used as these can exacerbate brain oedema.

Blood transfusion

Blood losses are generally small but massive losses can occur. Good venous access is required with the ability to transfuse large quantities of blood and colloid. Adequate fluid warming is important and access to blood and blood products at short notice is essential.

Measuring blood loss in paediatric neurosurgery is difficult and accurate blood replacement is only possible by careful clinical assessment of intravascular volume and by serial measurements of haematocrit. The Hb/PCV level at which red cell transfusion is triggered is discussed elsewhere.

Position

Ensure pressure points are protected and excessive traction on nerves such as the brachial plexus is avoided.

Supine

The majority of intracranial surgery occurs with the patient supine with the head turned to one side. It is important to ensure optimum venous drainage so a degree of 'head-up' tilt is desirable ($\pm 30°$) and, if the head is turned, jugular compression should be prevented.

Prone

Some intracranial surgery (e.g. posterior fossa) requires the patient to be positioned prone. It is important to avoid pressure on the abdomen which will increase the CVP and, thus, cerebral venous pressure. Pillows or other bolsters are used to support the pelvis and the chest to leave the abdomen free from compression.

Sitting

Use of the sitting position is controversial. The major concern is the possibility of air embolism. A recent large retrospective study of nearly 500 patients showed a 10% incidence of air embolism. If air embolism occurred, there was rarely any disturbance in cardiovascular variables. In addition, no morbidity could be attributed to air embolism in this study. The low incidence of air embolism in children is a result of less negative intracranial venous pressure compared with adults.

Hypotension is rarely a problem in children in the sitting position. The advantages of the sitting position include better surgical conditions and anatomical orientation, less bleeding, lower ICP and a lower incidence of postoperative cranial nerve damage.

Air embolism

Air embolism is a potential risk during any neurosurgical operation but particularly if the operative site is above the level of the heart. The dural venous sinuses are held open by the bone of the skull allowing entrainment of air.

Early recognition and treatment are the key to avoiding serious complications from air embolism.

Clinical signs of air embolism, in order of sensitivity, are:

- Changes in the precordial Doppler. This is a very sensitive monitor which may have limited effectiveness because of false positives.

- Sudden reduction in end-tidal CO_2 concentration.
- Reduction in S_aO_2.
- Cardiovascular changes – arrhythmias and hypotension.
- A machinery murmur can be heard if a precordial or oesophageal stethoscope is used ('mill-wheel' murmur).
- Cardiac arrest.

The most useful clinical indicator is a decrease in $ETCO_2$.
Management of air embolism includes:

- Inform the surgeon who floods the wound with saline.
- Call for help.
- Immediate pressure on the neck veins to increase CVP.
- Ventilate with 100% oxygen.
- Intravenous fluid bolus.

Prompt action will usually prevent further air entrainment and major haemodynamic problems but cardiopulmonary resuscitation may be required. Attempts to aspirate air from a central venous catheter should only be made after other treatment measures, as it is only successful in a few patients.

Postoperative care
- It is usually possible to extubate the trachea at the end of surgery. Postoperative ventilation may be necessary in some cases. Occasionally, continued ventilation may be required to protect the airway if a bulbar palsy has occurred.
- Patients should be cared for in a high-dependency/intensive care unit (ICU) by skilled neurosurgical nursing staff. It is usually necessary to continue invasive monitoring with assessment of conscious level, fluid balance and blood administration.
- Analgesia is usually with a combination of paracetamol and non-steroidal anti-inflammatory agents. Many centres still use codeine phosphate either rectally or orally. Some prefer nurse or patient-controlled analgesia with morphine or a simple morphine infusion.

Anaesthetic management of specific neurosurgical procedures
Hydrocephalus
Hydrocephalus and its surgical management is common in paediatric neurosurgery.

Classification of hydrocephalus
Congenital:
- Arnold–Chiari malformatiom
- myelomenigocele
- stenosis of the aqueduct
- idiopathic.

Acquired:
- infection
- intraventicular haemorrhage
- tumour.

The most common operation to treat hydrocephalus is a ventriculo-peritoneal shunt (V-P shunt). Occasionally, the ventricles are drained to the atrium or to the pleual space. Recently, it has become possible to use endoscopic ventriculoscopy to treat some forms of hydrocephalus. This involves the creation of a hole between ventricles allowing CSF to drain without the need for a shunt. This is a major advantage as the common complications of infection and blockage are avoided.

Anaesthetic considerations
- If the ICP is acutely raised, the patient may have been vomiting, become dehydrated and need IV fluid preoperatively.
- Conscious level may be reduced and in the presence of vomiting, pulmonary aspiration is a risk.
- Neurological status should be carefully monitored as rapid deterioration can occur.
- Sedative premedication is omitted. Local anaesthetic creams are useful for IV induction if a cannula is not in place.
- Surgery is frequently on very small expremature babies who have bronchopulmonary dysplasia and may be oxygen dependent. An ICU bed should be available if postoperative ventilation is required.
- Temperature maintenance is a problem, particularly in small babies having V-P shunts.
- Intubate with an armoured tracheal tube, and controlled ventilation.
- Significant blood loss is uncommon, and invasive monitoring is not usually required.
- Fentanyl 1–3 μg/kg is given before tunnelling the V-P catheter.
- Most children can be extubated at the end of anaesthesia, but should be cared for in a high-dependency neurosurgical area.
- Postoperative pain relief is with local anaesthesia to the abdominal wound, simple analgesics and codeine phosphate.

Craniopharyngioma

This is a tumour of the pituitary which causes visual disturbances because of pressure on the optic chiasma and also has endocrine effects, commonly panhypopituitarism. The endocrine effects may be present preoperatively or may occur during or after surgery. The surgical approach is via a frontal craniotomy.

Important clinical effects of panhypopituitarism include:

- adrenal insufficiency
- reduced growth hormone
- reduced thyroid hormone
- diabetes incipidus.

Anaesthetic considerations

- The child may be on corticosteroids or other replacement therapy including 1-deamino-8-D-argine vasopressin (DDAVP). The specialist advice of the endocrine team should be sought with regard to fluid and hormone replacement.
- Monitoring must include CVP, arterial cannula and urinary catheter.
- The ability to measure urine specific gravity and plasma osmolality perioperatively is essential.

Diabetes incipidus (DI)

DI occurs in craniopharyngioma but may also result from other intracranial pathology such as head injury, infection or tumours. As a result of a reduced or absent production of antidiuretic hormone, the kidney is unable to concentrate urine, which results in a large volume of dilute urine being excreted. Untreated, this rapidly results in dehydration and hypernatraemia.

The diagnosis of Dl is made if:

- urine output > 5 ml/kg/h
- urine specific gravity < 1005
- plasma osmolality > 290 mosmol/l.

Treatment includes:

- Management in high-dependency neurosurgical area
- Hourly urine output, urine specific gravity and regular plasma sodium and osmolality

- Maintenance fluid estimations – 0.45% saline
- Replace 3/4 previous hourly urine output with 0.45% saline
- DDAVP (desmopressin) 0.4 µg IM or intranasal.

Neural tube defects, meningomyelocoele and encephalocoele

The incidence is about 4 in 1000 live births. Meningomyelocoele is much more common than encephalocoele.

The spectrum of this defect is very large. Some lesions are completely covered with skin and barely detectable with very mild neurological signs, while others are very large lesions with a flimsy covering and associated with severe neurological impairment.

The urgency of closure of the lesion depends primarily on the risk of infection. In severe cases, surgery should take place as soon after delivery as possible. Surgical correction aims to cover the defect with skin and excise the sac. Hydrocephalus occurs in over 80% of patients with menigomyelocoele.

Anaesthetic considerations

- Surgery takes place on neonates. They are frequently small for dates or expremature. All aspects of neonatal anaesthesia apply.
- Careful assessment of the state of hydration is required. In severe lesions, large amounts of fluid may be lost. The defect is frequently covered with clear plastic drapes preoperatively.
- Positioning the patient for induction and intubation is difficult if the lesion is large. It is often necessary to support the baby on bolsters to take pressure off the lesion, and allow the baby to lie horizontally.
- Surgery takes place in the prone position. An armoured tracheal tube is required, with controlled ventilation and careful positioning to minimize abdominal pressure.
- Maintenance of body temperature is important, but difficult. Overhead radiant heaters, warm air devices and fluid warmers are necessary.
- Large blood losses can occur. Good venous access is needed and an arterial cannula is inserted for pressure monitoring and blood gas analysis. A central venous catheter is not indicated.
- Antibiotics are required.
- At the end of surgery, the trachea can usually be extubated but the baby requires postoperative care in a high-dependency area.
- Postopertive analgesia is with paracetamol and IV morphine.

13

Medical problems with particular relevance to paediatric anaesthesia

This chapter provides a brief outline of the more common paediatric conditions that have particular relevance to anaesthesia.

Respiratory conditions
Upper respiratory tract infection (URTI)
A common dilemma for paediatric anaesthetists is whether to postpone the patient with an upper respiratory tract infection. URTI is common in children and some almost always have a runny nose. It is not appropriate to defer all these children.

URTI causes an increase in perioperative complications including laryngospasm, bronchospasm, atelectasis and more rapid desaturation during apnoea. The risk is increased if the child is < 1 year old or is undergoing major surgery.

Elective surgery should be deferred if any of the following features are present:

- fever
- general malaise
- productive cough
- purulent secretions
- poor appetite
- chest signs
- know asthmatic child
- child < 1 year old
- major surgery.

If emergency surgery is required, airway problems should be anticipated.

Surgery should be deferred for 4 weeks after recovery from the illness as the complications associated with URTI are long lasting.

Asthma

Asthma is increasingly common, affecting approximately 1 : 10 children. Asthma may be triggered or exacerbated by URTI.

Childhood asthma is characterized by reversible airway obstruction with intermittent wheeze, difficulty in breathing, shortness of breath, cough and a feeling of tightness in the chest.

Precipitating factors include:

- URTI
- exercise
- allergy
- emotion
- cold air.

Mild asthma is extremely common and rarely requires extra precautions.

Anaesthesia

- Determine the severity of the asthma and ensure treatment is optimal.
- Defer if wheezing or URTI is present.
- Bronchodilators should be given before induction.
- Sedative premedication reduces anxiety.
- Avoid histamine-releasing drugs in severe asthma.
  - atracurium
  - thiopentone
  - morphine
  - succinylcholine.
- Propofol, vecuronium, rocuronium and fentanyl are preferable. Ketamine is a good bronchodilator.
- Intubation should be avoided if possible as it may precipitate bronchospasm.
- If intubation is required, ensure an adequate depth of anaesthesia.
- Humidification of inspired gases reduces the tenacity of secretions.
- Give supplementary hydrocortisone if the child has been taking oral steroids.

Management of bronchospasm during anaesthesia

Management includes:

- Deepen anaesthesia with volatile agents.

- Nebulize salbutamol into breathing circuit. For mild or moderate bronchospasm, use salbutamol 0.5% solution 0.5–1.0 ml diluted to 2 ml with saline. For severe bronchospasm, use undiluted solution.
- Intravenous salbutamol; 0.2–4 μg/kg/min (3 mg/kg in 50 ml 5% dextrose, 1 ml/h = 1 μg/kg/min).
- Adrenaline (epinephrine) IV bolus: 0.1–1.0 μg/kg. May be repeated or followed with an infusion: 0.01–0.1 μg/kg/min (300 μg/kg in 50 ml 5% dextrose, 1 ml/h = 0.1 μg/kg/min).
- Steroids
  - hydrocortisone 2–5 mg/kg IV
  - methylprednisolone 1 mg/kg.

Cystic fibrosis (CF)

Cystic fibrosis is inherited as an autosomal recessive condition that predominately affects the lungs but also affects the bowel, pancrease, biliary tract and sweat glands. The primary abnormality is in the chloride channel which leads to a high level of chloride in the sweat but which also causes abnormal mucus production in the lungs and is associated with abnormal ciliary activity. Medical treatment of CF has improved dramatically, resulting in improved life expectancy. Some children will require lung or heart–lung transplantation.

Pulmonary effects of CF are:

- chronic cough and wheeze
- production of copious, thick, abnormal secretions
- small airway obstruction with atalectasis
- recurrent infection (*pseudomonas aeruginosa* and *staphyococcus aureus*) with pneumonia, bronchiectasis and lung abscess
- V/Q mismatch with hypoxaemia
- risk of pneumothorax
- secondary right heart failure.

Other effects may include:

- meconium ileus (neonatal)
- poor nutritional state
- pancreatic insufficiency with hyperglycaemia
- portal hypertension and oesophageal varices
- malabsorption

Medical management of CF:

- physiotherapy
- antibiotics
- bronchodilators
- steroids
- pancreatic enzyme replacement
- nutritional supplementation

Anaesthesia
- Close liaison with the respiratory team for preoperative optimization of respiratory function.
- Preoperative physiotherapy and antibiotics.
- Continue routine medication.
- Avoid drying agents.
- Intubation is almost always required. Inflation pressures may be high.
- Minimize airway pressure to reduce risk of pneumothorax.
- Physiotherapy after intubation with tracheal suction is helpful. Request physiotherapy assistance in the operating room if necessary.
- Ensure good humidification of inspired gases and adequate hydration with IV fluids.
- Good postoperative analgesia to allow uninhibited coughing. Use regional analgesia where possible.
- Postoperative care with oxygen therapy, physiotherapy and good analgesia. Ventilation may be required in some cases. Intensive care requirements should be anticipated.

Bronchopulmonary dysplasia

Bronchopulmonary dysplasia (BPD) is a chronic lung disease of infancy which frequently follows neonatal respiratory distress syndrome. It is most common in expremature, low birth weight infants who required high inspired oxygen concentrations and pulmonary ventilation in the neonatal period. BPD is a major cause of morbitity and mortality.

Clinical features of BPD include:

- oxygen requirement after first month of life
- stiff lungs
- bronchoconstriction
- recurrent chest infections
- failure to thrive

- pulmonary hypertension and right heart failure
- reversion to a transitional circulation with right-to-left shunting secondary to pulmonary hypertension
- systemic hypertension
- chest X-ray changes include:
  - perihilar opacification
  - overexpansion with strands of opacification.

Management of BPD:

- supplementary oxygen or mechanical ventilation
- bronchodilators
- steroids
- diuretics
- nutritional support
- antibiotics when indicated.

Anaesthetic implications
- Respiratory assessment is focused on:
  - degree of respiratory support
  - current medication
  - clinical condition.
- Optimize pulmonary and cardiac function.
- Anticipate high inflation pressures and possibility of pneumothorax.
- Bronchospasm is common.
- Acute worsening of pulmonary hypertension is a risk.
- Development of a transitional circulation leads to hypoxia.
- Extubation is frequently problematic as on wakening from anaesthesia, coughing can precipitate bronchospasm, pulmonary hypertension and cyanosis.
- Postoperative respiratory complications are more common, including pneumothorax, atelectasis and chest infection.

Haematological disorders
Haemoglobin concentration and anaesthesia
The safe haemoglobin concentration (Hb) at which any child can be anaesthetized depends on the general condition of that child. For example, a child with stable chronic renal failure may only have an Hb of 7–8 g/dL but is quite accustomed to this degree of anaemia and can be safely anaesthetized. However, children with significant systemic

disease, particularly cardiac or respiratory disease, require a higher Hb as do premature infants (see Box 13.1).

Most children who are anaemic on routine screening have iron deficiency anaemia. Whether this is treated with iron supplements and dietary advice before elective surgery or not does not affect the incidence of perioperative complications.

Box 13.1   Normal haemoglobin concentrations in children

Age	Hb (g/dl)
Neonate	17–18
3 months	10–12
1 year	10–11
2 years	11–12
5 years	13
10 years	13–14

In otherwise healthy children, Hb of approximately 7.0 g/dl is usually accepted before a blood transfusion is considered.

Sickle cell disease

Sickle cell disease is an inherited condition caused by the substitution of valine for glutamic acid on the β-globin molecule. The resultant abnormal haemoglobin S (HbS) has a tendency to distort the red cell, forming a sickle shape when deoxygenated. This leads to haemolysis and sludging which occludes small vessels causing infarction and pain.

The disease occurs predominantly in people of Afro-Caribbean descent but also in those from the Mediterranean, Middle East or Indian subcontinent where it confers some protection against malaria.

The heterozygote form of sickle disease is known as sickle cell trait (HbAS), is usually asymptomatic and carries no significant anaesthetic implications. However, other abnormal haemoglobins such as HbC, HbD, HbE or β-thallasaemia may also occur in combination with HbS and this situation is more serious with a higher risk of sickling. The homozygous form HbSS, produces sickle cell disease and the severity of the disease depends on the percentage of HbS present. In neonates the high level of HbF is protective and affected infants do not manifest the disease until the HbF levels fall after the first few months of life.

Haemolysis causes an increase in the reticulocyte count and serum bilirubin. Acute severe haemolysis is known as a sickle crisis and may be precipitated by hypoxia, dehydration, acidosis or cold and results in severe pain. Apart from this haemolytic crisis, other acute complications occur including splenic autoinfarction, acute chest syndrome, overwhelming sepsis, aplasic anaemia and stroke. The skin can be affected by the vaso-occlusive nature of the disease as can the bone and other abdominal organs causing severe pain. Renal damage occurs as a result of repeated small infarcts.

The 'Sickledex' test is used as a screening test for sickle cell disease and a negative result confirms the absence of HbS. A positive test confirms the presence of HbS but does not distinguish between sickle trait and other forms of sickle cell disease. For definitive diagnosis and characterization of the haemoglobin, electrophoresis is required. Other useful laboratory tests are a full blood count, reticulocyte count and a peripheral blood film.

General management of patients with sickle cell disease includes:

- analgesia
- hydration
- blood transfusion
- bone marrow transplantation.

Anaesthetic implications and management
Children at risk of sickle cell disease should be screened preoperatively using the 'Sickledex' test which, if positive, is followed by a haemoglobin electrophoresis. Patients with HbAS (sickle trait) require no extra care.

Patients with sickle cell disease (HbSS):

- Involve a haematologist in the perioperative management.
- Transfusion: Traditional teaching has been to reduce levels of HbS to < 30–50% in patients who are symptomatic or who require major surgery. This necessitates exchange transfusions to increase the level of HbA and reduce the levels of HbS. Recently, it has been suggested that simple transfusion to 10 g/dl can reduce the risks of sickling during anaesthesia as effectively as exchange transfusion. This more conservative approach also decreases the risk of transfusion related complications. Patients who are well and having minor operations do not require transfusion.
- Hydration: Maintenance IV fluids should be given during the period of starvation and throughout surgery to avoid dehydration. In addi-

tion, careful intravascular fluid replacement should be undertaken to avoid hypovolaemia.
- Avoid hypoxia.
- Maintain body temperature.
- Effective analgesia.

Thallasaemia

Thallasaemia is an inherited disease affecting haemoglobin synthesis, either the α- or β-globin chain. Thallasaemia occurs mainly in Mediterranean, African or Asian people.

α-Thallasaemia

There is a broad spectrum of disease depending on the number of genes (1–4) involved. With a single gene, patients are asymptomatic but with two genes a moderate anaemia is present. When three genes are involved, a severe haemolytic anaemia with jaundice and splenomegaly develops, and with four abnormal genes the disease is usually fatal.

β-Thallasaemia

This is classified as either minor or major depending on whether one or two genes are abnormal. In β-thallasaemia major, children develop haemolytic anaemia in the first few months of life which is treated by repeated blood transfusion. The risk of iron overload is reduced if a chelating agent such as desferrioxamine is used. An increasing number of these patients are now treated with bone marrow transplantation. β thallasaemia minor is very mild and children are asymptomatic or may have a mild hypochromic, microcytic anaemia.

Anaesthetic implications are limited to ensuring an adequate Hb before surgery. Those patients with HbS-thallasaemia should be managed in the same manner as those with sickle cell disease.

Haemophilia

Haemophilia is an X-linked recessive disorder that affects 1: 10 000 boys. Haemophilia A results from a factor VIII deficiency and is four times more common than haemophilia B which results from a factor IX deficiency. The clinical presentation of haemophilia A and B is identical and the severity of the disease depends on the levels of factor VIII or IX in the plasma. Neonatal presentation may be with bleeding from the umbilicus or after circumcision.

Bleeding depends on the severity of disease:

- Mild (factor levels 5–50 IU/dl): Bleeding generally noticed only after trauma or surgery.
- Moderate (factor levels 1–5 IU/dl): Spontaneous soft tissue haematomas and mucosal bleeds.
- Severe (factor levels < 1 IU/dl): Spontaneous bleeding into muscle, joints and also intracranial, gastrointestinal and retroperitoneal bleeds.

Coagulation profiles in haemophilia:

- prothrombin time (PT) normal
- activated partial thromboplastin time (APTT) prolonged
- platelet count normal
- bleeding time normal
- specific factor levels reduced (VIII or IX).

Management involves:

- Replacement of specific factors to prevent major bleeding and chronic joint damage caused by repeated haemarthroses.
- If bleeding occurs, replacement specific factors are given to increase factor activity:
  - minor bleeding ↑ 30%
  - moderate bleeding ↑ 50%
  - major bleeding ↑ 100%.
- 1-deamino-8-D-arginine vasopressin (DDAVP/desmopressin) is also given as it increases the levels of factor VIII.

Anaesthetic management
- These children are best managed in cooperation with a haematologist with a special interest in haemophilia.
- The aim of preoperative management is to give sufficient clotting factors to increase activity levels to reduce intra- or postoperative bleeding.
- The factor activity levels required for surgery are:
  - for minor superficial surgery 50%
  - for major surgery 100%
  - postoperatively keep levels between 25–100% for 10 days.

von Willibrand's disease

This autosomal dominant condition is the most common inherited coagulopathy and may affect up to 1% of children. The basic defect is the abnormal synthesis of a glycoprotein, known as von Willibrand's factor (vWF), which is required for the normal function of platelets and factor VIII. It has been classified into three types.

Classification:

- Type I, mild:
  Most common, 90% of affected children. Bruising after trauma or surgery or mild mucosal bleeding such as epistaxis.
- Type II, moderate:
  Spontaneous mucosal, skin or gastrointestinal bleeding can occur. A subgroup can also have thrombocytopenia.
- Type III, severe:
  Severe bleeding with joints affected.

Diagnosis:

- bleeding time is generally prolonged
- APTT is prolonged but PT and TT are usually normal
- vWF is assayed for definitive diagnosis.

Management includes:

- DDAVP (vasopressin)
- vWF concentrate.

Anaesthetic management
- A haematologist should be involved.
- Patients with type I and II having minor surgery are given DDAVP.
- Patients with type III having minor or major surgery or types I and II having major surgery should be given vWF.
- Failure of intraoperative haemostasis should be treated with a platelet transfusion.

Malignant disease

Leukaemia

Leukaemia accounts for 50% of all childhood malignancy. The majority of leukaemias are acute, either acute lymphoblastic leukaemia (ALL) or acute myeloid leukaemia (AML). A minority are chronic, usually chronic myeloid leukaemia (CML).

Lymphoma

Hodgkin's lymphoma

This presents as painless swelling of the lymph nodes and diagnosis is made on biopsy. These patients may have large mediastinal masses which may compromise the airway during anaesthesia. The majority of patients are treated with chemotherapy but radiotherapy is also used.

Non-Hodgkin's lymphoma

This usually presents with an abdominal mass arising from enlargement of abdominal lymphoid tissue. Classification is into lymphoblastic and non-lymphoblastic (Burkitt's lymphoma). Treatment is with chemotherapy but the prognosis is less good than Hodgkin's lymphoma.

Anaesthetic implications of malignant disease

The anaesthetist may be involved in the care of patients with malignant disease, either in surgery to remove solid tumour, or during investigation (lumbar puncture, bone marrow aspirate), or for central line insertion.

There are a number of common effects of malignant disease and its treatment which are of relevance during anaesthesia:

- Infection is a constant threat in the immunocompromised child and careful aseptic technique is required.
- Clotting abnormalities can result from a low platelet count as well as other causes.
- Chemotherapeutic agents may cause liver damage or cardiomyopathy.
- Pancytopenia may be part of the disease or a result of chemotherapy. Blood or blood products may need to be given. Irradiated or leucocyte-depleted products should be used to prevent graft-versus-host disease.
- Massive tumour necrosis may occur at the onset of treatment. This leads to high circulating levels of uric acid and phosphate, which cause renal failure. Allopurinol and hyperhydration is used to reduce this risk, but fluid overload can result leading to pulmonary oedema.
- Tumour mass can exert an effect at any anatomical site. Masses in the anterior mediastinum are dangerous as they can cause airway or superior vena cava obstruction. Airway obstruction is a particular problem after induction of anaesthesia as, with the loss of compensating muscle tone, the trachea or main bronchi may be occluded.

Careful preoperative assessment must include a search for stridor or other respiratory compromise, including any worsening of symptoms on changes in position, and a review of X-rays and magnetic resonance imaging/computed tomography scans to show the extent of the mass. A rigid bronchoscope should be prepared before induction so that if airway collapse occurs the bronchoscope can provide a temporary airway. An inhalational induction is advisable and, if possible, a spontaneous breathing technique should be used. If obstruction occurs during anaesthesia a change in position may be helpful.

Other considerations:

- Massive hepatosplenomegaly can cause abdominal swelling and compromise breathing.
- When using tunnelled, central venous cathethers (Hickman, PICC) ensure a no-touch or aseptic technique is used. Any channel that is used should be flushed carefully with 20 ml saline or heparin-saline.

Diabetes mellitus

Diabetes mellitus is the most common endocrine disease in children and is usually Type I (insulin dependent) diabetes.

Clinical features:

- polydipsia
- polyuria
- weight loss
- hyperglycaemia
- glycosuria
- ketosis

The long-term complications of diabetes are seldom seen in children, but childhood diabetes tends to be unstable metabolically and diabetic ketoacidosis is a risk. Diabetic ketoacidosis may mimic an acute abdomen, but ketoacidosis is more common in those with an acute systemic illness, including surgical emergencies.

Anaesthetic management

- The aim of perioperative management is to maintain blood glucose levels as close to normal as possible. Input from the diabetic team is helpful.
- Perioperative protocols vary, but involve the infusion of glucose, insulin and potassium.

For short procedures, where the child is expected to drink and eat very soon after surgery, an infusion of glucose and insulin is unnecessary.

- Omit breakfast
- give 1/2 normal insulin
- check glucose hourly
- restart normal insulin when eating.

Perioperative management of children with diabetes undergoing lengthy surgical procedures:

- Admit the child the day before surgery.
- Schedule the child first on the operating list the following morning.
- Check blood glucose and electrolytes.
- Rapid-acting insulin before supper (no long- or intermediate-acting insulin).
- Start infusion at bedtime or 4 h after supper, whichever comes sooner:
  - 500 ml 10% glucose and 0.18% sodium chloride solution
  - add 10 mmol potassium chloride
  - add soluble insulin 12 units
  - This should run at 50 ml/kg per 24 h.

If surgery is scheduled to take place in the afternoon then give breakfast with rapid-acting insulin and start infusion 4 h later.

Blood glucose should be checked 2-hourly before surgery and hourly during surgery.

- If blood glucose is > 10 mmol/l increase insulin to 16 units per 500 ml infusion bag.
- If blood glucose is < 5 mmol/l reduce insulin to 8 units per 500 ml infusion bag.
- Infusion should be continued until eating is restarted, when usual insulin given.

Mucopolysaccharidoses

This is a group of disorders in which the primary abnormality is the deposition of mucopolysaccharides in various body tissue. They are all inherited as recessive traits except for Hunter's disease, which is X-linked. They are classified from I to VII. Prenatal diagnosis is possible and treatment for some types (Hunter's and Hurler's) is with bone marrow transplantation which, although not curative, usually halts its progression.

Hurler's syndrome (Type I) presents in the first year of life with an increase in head size, coarse facies and small stature. Associated features include short neck, corneal clouding, mental retardation, hydrocephalus, deafness and scoliosis resulting in a restrictive lung disorder. Cardiomyopathy or valve disease is usually the cause of death in the first decade without bone marrow transplantation.

Hunter's syndrome (Type II) is similar to Type I with dwarfism, coarse features, corneal clouding, cardiac involvement and hydrocephalus but in addition retinitis pigmentosa may be present.

The implications for anaesthesia include:

- Obstructive sleep apnoea.
- Difficult airway due to abnormal mucopolysaccharide deposition in the tissues. Airway compromise worsens with age if no treatment is given. It is often possible to manage this difficult airway with an LMA™ but tracheostomy may be required.
- The intubation may be very difficult or impossible. A fibreoptic bronchoscope may be useful.
- Cardiac involvement with cardiomyopathy and valve disease means that a cardiology assessment before anaesthesia is necessary.
- Restrictive lung disease.

Other types include Sanfilippo's (III), Morquio's (IV) with neck instability, Maroteaux–Lamy (VI) and Sly (VII) – all may cause difficulties with the airway.

Down's syndrome (trisomy 21)

Down's syndrome is relatively common occurring in 1–2 per 1000 live births. These children have characteristic facies, a complete palmer crease, microcephaly, macroglossia and hypotonia. Congenital heart disease also occurs, particularly atrioventricular septal defect, ventricular septal defect, patent ductus arteriosus and tetralogy of Fallot. Atlanto-axial instability is frequently a problem and a cervical X-ray in both flexion and extension should be obtained before anaesthesia if there is any suggestion of neurological involvement. Congenital subglottic stenosis may be present and, even in its absence, post-intubation stridor is more common.

Anaesthesia

- Potentially difficult airway because of large tongue.
- Avoid extension of neck because of risk of atlanto-axial subluxation (20% of children with Down's syndrome).

- Select a smaller tracheal tube and ensure a leak is present to reduce the risk of post-intubation stridor. Steroids decrease laryngeal oedema after prolonged intubation.
- A careful preoperative cardiac evaluation is required. Antibiotic prophylaxis may be indicated.
- Increased sensitivity to muscle relaxants and volatile agents.
- Difficult peripheral venous access.
- More difficult to place internal jugular catheter because of indistinct landmarks. Extra care is required with positioning because of the dangers of potential neck instability.
- Developmental delay makes the children less able to cooperate with induction of anaesthesia.

Latex allergy

Latex allergy (allergy to natural rubber) is a problem for patients and for health professionals. Latex is obtained from the rubber tree *Hevea brasiliensis* and the allergy is usually IgE mediated.

Risk factors for latex allergy:

- multiple operations
- history of myelodysplasia
- neurogenic bladder
- genitourinary abnormalities, particularly bladder extrophy
- atopy with asthma or eczema
- food allergy (banana, avocado, kiwi fruit, chestnuts)
- facial swelling with balloons.

Latex allergy is the most common cause of anaphylaxis during anaesthesia in children and may account for 70% of all reactions. The incidence of sensitization (RAST IgE positive) to latex is about 6–10% of children presenting for surgery in the UK. Only a small proportion of these go on to develop anaphylaxis during anaesthesia, but when they do occur these reactions are life threatening. The onset of anaphylaxis may be gradual, so diagnosis can be delayed, and the severity also varies widely.

The signs of latex allergy during anaesthesia include:

- bronchospasm with increased airway pressure
- hypotension
- tachycardia

- decreases in oxygen saturation
- periorbital or facial swelling
- urticaria and rash.

Prophylaxis against latex allergy is defined as primary or secondary. Primary prophylaxis is designed to prevent patients from developing latex sensitization and secondary prophylaxis prevents anaphylaxis occurring in those already sensitized. The only reliable strategy for primary prophylaxis is to make hospitals latex-free environments with particular emphasis on latex-free gloves. Secondary prophylaxis is well established in many hospitals with 'latex allergy' protocols. The basis of any protocol is the avoidance of latex. A list of latex-free products should be available and a latex-free anaesthetic trolley should be available. There is controversy about the use of drug prophylaxis. Some argue that it is useful in reducing the severity of reactions when they occur while others maintain that it decreases neither the incidence nor severity of reactions, is expensive, has potential risks and may extend the hospital stay.

The following regimen is suggested:

- methylprednisolone 1 mg/kg 6 h IV (maximum dose 50 mg per dose)
- ranitidine 1 mg/kg IV slowly 6 h.
- Chlorpheniramine
  - < 1 years 250 µg/kg IV 6 h
  - 1–5 years 2.5–5 mg IV 6 h
  - 6–12 years 5–10 mg IV 6 h
  - >12 years 10–20 mg IV 6 h.

At least two doses of each of these should be given preoperatively.

The child should be scheduled first on the list to reduce the levels of aero-allergens, and signs should be placed on the operating room door and on the patients notes and bed. Care should be taken not to draw up drugs through rubber bungs or inject through rubber bungs on the IV giving sets.

Treatment of a reaction depends on the severity but should be primarily with adrenaline (epinephrine). Initially, a small bolus of adrenaline (epinephrine) 0.1–1 µg/kg should be used (NB 10–100 µg/kg during cardiac arrest). This can be followed by an adrenaline (epinephrine) infusion 0.1–0.3 µg/kg/min.

Other measures include those that would be given for any anaphylaxis:

- Volume replacement 10 ml/kg bolus
- 100% oxygen
- steroids: hydrocortisone 2–5 mg/kg
- Chlorpheniramine
- Ranitide 1 mg/kg slowly.

Anaesthesia in children post-transplantation

Organ transplantation is increasingly successful in children, who will often present for surgery for unrelated conditions.

Important considerations include:

- Immunosuppression therapy, evidence of rejection.
- Steroid use, additional steroids may be needed.
- Increased risk of infection.
- Evidence of other organ effects of drug regimen, e.g. renal damage, clotting abnormalities.
- Psychological stress may be increased in the child and family.
- Liason with the principal care team.

Cardiac transplantation

- Cardiac review, assessment of function.
- Rejection is manifested as pyrexia, lethargy, electrocardiogram (ECG) changes and subtle decrease in cardiac function on echocardiography (ECHO). These symptoms may masquerade as acute illness and it is important to ensure rejection is not occurring, as surgery undertaken during rejection is poorly tolerated.
- Isoprenaline is the drug of choice for bradycardia, as the heart is denervated.
- Use monitoring appropriately and preserve access points such as the internal jugular vein as this is needed long-term for endomyocardial biopsy.
- Coronary arteriosclerosis is common in the transplanted heart and painless ischaemia may be present.
- Check ECG. Sudden death from coronary occlusion occurs. Post-transplant protocols include routine coronary angiography.

Renal transplantation

- Assessment of renal function. A well-functioning transplanted kidney will result in normal basic renal function tests.
- Avoid non-steroidal anti-inflammatory drugs.

- Maintain an adequate blood pressure. Ensure good renal perfusion.
- Avoid placing vascular cannulae in sites that may be useful for arteriovenous shunts in the future.

Children post-cardiac surgery who present for non-cardiac surgery

All children require assessment of their present status and consideration of the need for antibiotic prophylaxis.

In many instances, cardiac surgery has resulted in a structurally and functionally normal heart. In this case, the child will be having yearly cardiology reviews and information from their last review is sufficient for adequate assessment.

In other more complex cases, the child may have important differences in cardiac structure and/or function. This is assessed at a cardiology review which includes an ECHO and ECG. Important features to determine include:

- ventricular function
- presence of intracardiac mixing
- patency of surgically created shunts
- evidence of any right or left ventricular outflow tract obstruction.
- cyanosis
- polycythaemia, (secondary to cyanosis) which, if severe, is associated with increased viscosity, poor microperfusion and a risk of stroke and cerebral abscess.

Specific issues indicating high risk include:

- Polycythaemia, which may need to be treated by venesection. Additional IV fluids must be given and fasting minimized.
- Significant outflow tract obstruction, particularly of the left heart.
- Pulmonary hypertension.
- Poor ventricular function.
- Presence of a Fontan circulation. In children with complex repairs resulting in single-ventricle physiology (Fontan circulation), the heart is reliant on high right-sided venous pressures and cardiac filling must be optimized.

14

Local anaesthetic techniques

Whenever possible, local anaesthesia should be used to complement general anaesthesia (see Box 14.1).

Box 14.1 Advantages and disadvantages with local anaesthesia

Advantages	Disadvantages
Prolonged pain relief	Risk of infection
Early mobilization	Side effects of individual block (see below)
Decreased use of analgesics such as morphine	Potentially increased risk of nerve damage as usually performed under general anaesthesia
Less nausea and vomiting	Risk of agent toxicity
Decreased physiological response to surgery	
Lighter plane of anaesthesia required	

Common routes of administration include:

- topical
- local infiltration
- peripheral nerve blockade
- central nerve blocks, spinal, epidural.

Each technique has potential complications. If the anaesthetic plan includes use of a specific technique, it is important to discuss the risks and benefits of any block with the family and child, where appropriate. When local or central blockade is not suitable, simple wound infiltration often provides excellent analgesia for several hours postoperatively.

Contraindications to a local technique
- coagulopathy
- local or systemic infection

- local anatomical abnormality
- local neurological abnormality
- sensitivity to local anaesthetic agent
- patient refusal.

Local anaesthetic drugs
Maximum doses of local anaesthetic agents
Toxic effects of local anaesthetics are related to plasma concentrations. The maximum safe doses reflect a general guide only (see Box 14.2). Plasma level is affected by:

- The dose given.
- The site used, e.g. absorption from the epidural space is greater than from subcutaneous infiltration. Note: accidental intravascular injection is the main cause of toxicity.
- The use of adrenaline (epinephrine), particularly with lignocaine, which decreases absorption.
- Absorption, distribution and metabolism of the individual drug.

Box 14.2 Maximum recommended doses		
Drug	**Child (mg/kg)**	**Usual concentration %**
Bupivacaine	2.5	0.25, 0.5
Lignocaine	3 (plain)	0.5, 1.0
	7 (with epinephrine)	
Ropivacaine		0.2,
Prilocaine	5	0.5, 1.0, 2.0,
Levobupivacaine	2.5	0.25, 0.5

Toxicity of local anaesthetics
Most blocks in children are done following induction of general anaesthesia, so the early warning signs of toxicity described in adult practice are not seen. All patients should be monitored during induction and placement of blocks. Great care with dosage and performance of blocks is essential. Accidental intravascular injections must be avoided. If aspiration of blood occurs during placement of the block, the position of needle/catheter should be adjusted. Rarely, acute sensitivity to specific local anaesthetics may occur. Dysrhythmias, hypotension, convulsions or cardiac arrest may result from toxicity. Cardiac toxicity related to bupivacaine is particularly resistant to treatment. Paevobupi-

vacaine is safer. Rarely, acute sensitivity to specific local anaesthetics may occur.

Topical anaesthetic agents
Ametop
- 4% amethocaine (tetracaine).
- Not recommended in neonates or premature babies, as absorption is rapid with concern about potential toxicity.
- Skin reactions are common.
- Apply for at least 45 min.
- Do not leave longer than 1 h as burns have been reported following prolonged application.
- Anaesthesia lasts 4–5 h.

EMLA
- 1 ml contains 25 mg prilocaine and 25 mg lignocaine.
- Apply for at least 60 min.
- Skin reaction (less frequent than with ametop).
- Risk of methaemoglobinaemia if large amount used.
- Not recommended < 1 year due to concerns of toxicity. However, toxicity is unlikely provided use is confined to IV cannulation sites.

Box 14.3   Adjuncts to local anaesthetics

Drug	Dose	Common formulations	Used for
Adrenaline (epinephrine)	5–10 µg/kg	1 in 200 000 (5 µg/ml) 1 in 100 000 (10 µg/ml) 1 in 80 000 (12.5 µg/ml)	Most blocks except digital and penile
Clonidine	1–2 µg/kg		Caudal/epidural
Morphine	20 to 100 µg/kg		Caudal/epidural
Fentanyl	1–2 µg/ kg		Caudal/epidural
Ketamine	0.5 mg/ml		Caudal/epidural

NB: Drugs used for epidural administration must be preservative free.

Adrenaline (epinephrine) (Box 14.3)
- Vasoconstrictor.
- Decreases vascular absorption, so more effective at the membrane.

- Prolongs the length of action of local anaesthesia. This effect is greatest with lignocaine and less so with bupivacaine, bupivacaine and ropivacaine.
- Used in a test dose to check intravascular injection has not occurred.

Clonidine
- used in caudals and epidurals
- prolongs analgesia × 2
- increased sedation
- may delay discharge for day cases
- hypotension can occur when used with caudal bupivacaine and so often avoided in day cases.

Ketamine
- adjunct to caudals and epidurals
- prolongs analgesia × 4
- may delay discharge for day cases.

Opiates, opioids, e.g. morphine, fentanyl
- used with caudal/epidural blocks
- increases and prolongs analgesia
- potential side effects include:
  - itching
  - nausea and vomiting
  - apnoea
  - delayed respiratory depression
  - urinary retention
- not used for day cases due to concerns about delayed respiratory depression.

Local anaesthetic blocks commonly used in paediatrics
An IV cannula is placed and routine monitoring established before starting any block. All local blocks are done with a sterile technique. Short bevelled needles are useful for identifying the tissue layers and are less traumatic to nerves. A nerve stimulator is useful in blocks, such as brachial plexus, to decrease the risk of damage to the nerves in the anaesthetized child.

Local infiltration
This is simple and can be done in most sites. Infiltration can be done before or after surgery. Care must be taken not to exceed the recommended maximum dose the drug used.

Subcutaneous infusions using a fine-bore catheter connected to a syringe pump are useful postoperatively. For example, in donor bone graft sites, bupivacaine 0.25% at 2–4 ml/h.

Topical anaesthetics

Topical EMLA or ametop are also useful for circumcision, biopsy or skin donor sites. Care must be taken to avoid application of excessive amounts either individually or on repeated use. Absorption of significant amounts of local anaesthetic can occur if large donor skin areas are treated. The onset of action is quicker with ametop than EMLA and vasodilatation more likely, but side effects, such as skin irritation, are greater.

Dental blocks

Used mainly by dentists to provide analgesia following dental extraction. The injection is done with infiltration in the buccal sulcus providing a block of the long buccal nerve. An inferior dental nerve block affects the lower teeth and half the lip. Infiltration of the buccal and palatal aspects of the palate provides analgesia for palate repairs. Infraorbital nerve blocks, either transcutaneously or sub-buccally, provide excellent analgesia for cleft lip repairs.

Use 1% lignocaine with adrenaline (epinephrine) 1 in 80 000 or 0.5% lignocaine with 1 in 200 000 adrenaline (epinephrine). Maximum recommended adrenaline (epinephrine) 10 µg/kg.

Infraorbital block

Provides good analgesia following repair of cleft lip

Equipment	23 or 25 G needle
Technique	Palpate the infraorbital groove, insert the needle perpendicularly to the skin to touch bone, and then withdraw a few millimetres. If the aspiration test is negative instill local anaesthetic.
Dose	0.5–0.75 ml 0.5% bupivacaine

Ilioinguinal L1, and iliohypogastric T12, L1 block

Indication: For hernia repair, hydrocele or orchidopexy

Position	Supine
Equipment	22 G needle or short bevelled needle

Site	Identify the anterior superior iliac spine. Insert the needle 1 cm medial and 1 cm inferior to this, advance feeling the 'pop' of the external and internal oblique fascia.
	Half the dose is given at this point and then the remainder in a fan shape area towards the iliac bone as the needle is withdrawn.
Dose	Large volumes are used – 0.25% bupivacaine 0.5–1.0 ml/kg. If bilateral blocks are done, do not exceed recommended doses.
Specific risks/ complications	Femoral nerve block occurs in approximately 10% resulting in leg weakness.

Dorsal penile nerve block, S2, 3, 4

Indication: For circumcision, meatotomy and distal hypospadias surgery

Position	Supine
Equipment	22 or 23 G needle
Site	a) place needle in the midline just inferior to the symphysis pubis, advance slowly, vertically, feeling the 'pop' as you pass Bucks fascia to instil the local anaesthetic. Aspirate frequently to avoid intravascular injection.
	b) a lateral approach uses two injection sites, both just below the pubis but each 0.5–1.0 cm away from the midline. Advance until you 'pop' through the fascia for instillation.
Dose	1.0–5.0 ml of 0.25% bupivacaine. *Adrenaline (epinephrine) must not be used* as local spasm of the dorsal penile arteries may result in ischaemia.
Specific complications	Risk of corpus cavernosum haematoma, particularly with the midline approach. The genital branch of the genitofemoral nerve supplies the base of the penis so the penile block is not used for

extensive hypospadias repairs when a caudal provides better analgesia.

Brachial plexus block, axillary approach

- safest approach to block the brachial plexus in children
- useful for hand and distal arm surgery.

Position	Supine with the shoulder abducted and the elbow flexed so that the hand can rest against the head.
Equipment	22 or 20 G cannula. A nerve stimulator can be used.
Technique	Palpate the axillary artery high in the axilla. Insert cannula and feel a click as it passes into the axillary sheath. The cannula will pass easily into the sheath. Aspirate and, if negative, instill the anaesthetic.
	Compress the arm below the injection point to prevent the drug from spreading down the sheath. An alternative method is to use a trans-arterial approach for the injection.
Dose	Large volumes are used, 0.5–1.0 ml/kg 0.25% bupivacaine
Complications	Block can have a prolonged effect lasting up to 24 h and the arm must be protected.

Great auricular nerve (GAN)

Indication: analgesia for the correction of bat ears (otoplasty)

Position	Supine with head rotated
Site	3 ml local anaesthetic is placed:
	anterior to the mastoid to block the anterior divisions of the GAN
	posterior to the mastoid to block the posterior divisions of the GAN
	anterior to the external auditory meatus to block the auriculotemporal nerve (a branch of the mandibular division of the trigeminal nerve).

Caudal

This is useful for abdominal (T9 and below), perineal and lower limb surgery. An initial bolus of bupivacaine provides 4–6 h of adequate analgesia. For longer duration, a caudal catheter may be placed and an infusion of local anaesthetic continued postoperatively. Catheter types and infusion regimens are similar to those used in epidural techniques. A caudal catheter inserted up to abdominal or thoracic levels is usually successful in smaller children and infants.

Position	Lateral, hips and knees flexed
Equipment	20–22 G needle or cannula, Tuohy needle (if a catheter is to be used), block needle.
Method	Identify the sacral cornua, insert needle between them into the sacrococcygeal space at 90° angle, then reposition needle to approximately 30° to the skin and advance towards the head until the caudal membrane is traversed. Check there is no aspiration of blood or cerebrospinal fluid (CSF). Inject local anaesthetic slowly, reaspirating part way through to ensure no aspiration of blood or CSF.
Dose	0.25% bupivacaine, volume depends on level of anaesthesia required: sacral 0.5 ml/kg inguinal/hip/lower limb 0.75 ml/kg abdominal 1.0 ml/kg. The duration of the block is extended with clonidine, ketamine or opiate (see above). In small babies a 0.2% solution can be made by diluting 4 ml of 0.25% bupivacaine with 1 ml saline and then using a maximum of 1 ml/kg.
Specific risks	Leg weakness is common, due to motor block
Complications	Dural puncture Haematoma Intravascular injection

| | Risk of burns if a leg is placed near a radiator whilst sensation is diminished. Urinary retention |
| Specific | Sacral abnormalities, spina bifida, previous spinal surgery |

Epidural

Indications: Major thoracic, abdominal, pelvic and lower limb surgery. A 'single-shot' epidural with bupivacaine will provide 4–6 h of analgesia. A catheter with infused local anaesthetic may be left in place for 2–3 days.

Method	These blocks must be done with full aseptic technique, gloves and face mask.
Position	Lateral, knees and hips flexed
Equipment	19 G Tuohy needle with 23 G catheter for use in infants up to approximately 10 kg and 18 G needle with a 21 G catheter above this weight. In children over 8 years of age 16g G Tuohy with an 18 G catheter may be used.
Site	Identify the midline of the intervertebral space (usually L2–3). Make a small skin incision, insert the Tuohy slowly into the ligamentum flavum, then advance using a saline-filled syringe to identify the loss of resistance when entering the epidural space. The distance from the skin to the epidural spaces can be estimated with various formulae using weight, surface area and age. A catheter is advanced to the required level; at least 4 cm should be left in the space. Fix carefully, as children move readily.
Doses	This depends on the sensory level to be blocked and the site of the catheter tip. 0.25% bupivacaine up to 0.75 ml/kg for abdominal or thoracic surgery. An infusion of 0.125% bupivacaine 0.1–0.4 ml/kg/h, adjusted as needed.

Specific risks	technical difficulties
Complications	dural tap
	haematoma
	infection, which can be superficial or deep
	hypotension (uncommon in young children)
	total spinal injection
	risks associated with opiates, if used
	urinary retention
	neurological damage (rare)

Spinal

Indications: Particularly in neonates for inguinal hernia repair or anorectal surgery taking approximately 1 h.

Associated with less risk of apnoea if used without sedation or general anaesthesia. Blood pressure is usually well maintained as small babies do not have high vascular tone, so autonomic blockade has little effect.

Position	Lateral, held carefully with the spine flexed
Equipment	24 or 22 G spinal needle
Site	Identify the interspinous space at L3/4 or L4/5, (the spinal cord reaches L3 in the neonate)
Method/Dose	0.5% bupivacaine 0.1 ml/kg
	0.5% heavy bupivacaine 0.1 ml/kg allow for the dead space of the needle
Complications	Failure rate 10%
	Little postoperative analgesia
	Risk of high block resulting in respiratory muscle weakness
	Dural puncture headache in older children

15

Management of trauma and transport of the paediatric patient

The injured child

Trauma is the commonest cause of death in children outside the neonatal period (see Box 15.1). Emergency management includes resuscitation and stabilization. Initially, a primary survey provides a rapid and systematic review. A subsequent secondary survey involves a thorough physical examination after resuscitation has been accomplished. It should be borne in mind that bleeding may be hidden.

In addition, all trauma patients require:

- Good vascular access.
- Hb, U&E, clotting and blood cross-match. Additional blood products will be required if massive transfusion is given.
- Nasogastric tube, gastric stasis and distension may occur; assume delayed stomach emptying when planning induction of anaesthesia.
- Antibiotic cover and review of tetanus immunization status.

Box 15.1   Aetiology of trauma

Babies	Children
Birth trauma	Road traffic accidents
Birth asphyxia	Accidents in the home, falls,
Shoulder dystrophia, brachial plexus damage	Non-accidental injury
Head injury	Accidental ingestion of drugs or poisons
	Thermal injury burns, hypothermia (core temperature < 35°C)

Assessment

Following any severe injury a child must be assessed systematically. Initially, a primary survey is used to identify any life threatening conditions.

Primary survey
- airway
- breathing
- circulation
- disability – neurological deficit
- exposure – thermal injury, (usually hypothermia).

Once the child has been adequately resuscitated, his/her condition is stable and they are monitored appropriately, a careful secondary survey is undertaken.

Secondary survey
- thorough examination
- history of injury
- previous medical history
- investigations, blood tests, X-rays, scans
- re evaluation and plan for further management.

Examination for damage related to
- head injury
- neck injury
- chest
- abdomen
- pelvis
- spine and limbs
- any skin damage.

Head injury

Head injury results in a primary injury that causes damage at the time, which is followed by secondary injury. The secondary injury is the later evolution of the injury resulting from hypoxia, cerebral oedema or hypotension. Blunt head trauma is more common than penetrating injury (stabbing or gunshot) in young patients. If intervention is rapid, secondary injury can be limited. Neurological outcome can be very good in the young even after severe trauma.

Assessment
Primary survey
A rapid systematic evaluation to assess airway, breathing and circulation to ensure these are adequate.

Determine the Glasgow Coma Score (GCS), which is slightly modified for use in paediatrics (see Box 15.2).

Box 15.2   Glasgow Coma Score in Children

Response	Children	Infants	Points
Eye opening	None	None	1
	To pain	To pain	2
	To voice	To voice	3
	Spontaneous	Spontaneous	4
Verbal	None	None	1
	Incomprehensible	Moaning	2
	Inappropriate words	Cries to pain	3
	Confused	Irritable	4
	Oriented	Babbling	5
Motor	None	None	1
	Decerebrate posturing	Decerebrate posturing	2
	Decorticate posturing	Decorticate posturing	3
	Withdraws to pain	Withdraws to pain	4
	Localises pain	Withdraws to touch	5
	Obeys commands	Normal movements	6

A total score is between 3 and 15. GCS ≤ 8 implies significant neurological damage has occurred. GCS ≤ 8 usually associated with airway difficulties and intubation is required (see Box 15.2).

Secondary survey

A careful general and neurological evaluation to look for in particular:

- head injury, results of X-ray, computed tomography (CT), magnetic resonance imaging
- neck injury, especially cervical spine to C7, using X-rays or CT
- evidence of base of skull fracture, e.g. cerebrospinal fluid leak from ear or nose
- maxillofacial fractures
- eyes and ears for injuries.

Chest trauma

- Blunt trauma (road traffic accidents, falls) is much commoner than penetrating injuries in children.
- Frequently associated with other significant injuries, e.g. head, abdominal trauma.
- Most chest injuries will not need surgery.

- May result in:
  - airway obstruction
  - pneumothorax, tension pneumothorax, haemopneumothorax
  - lung contusion
  - rib fractures, flail chest
  - myocardial contusion (electrocardiogram (ECG) changes, atrial or ventricular ectopics, dysrhythmias, ischaemia)
  - cardiac tamponade (increasing central venous pressure, decreased blood pressure, pulsus paradoxus; confirm with echocardiography, chest X-ray)
  - major vessel rupture, pulmonary vessels, aorta.

Abdominal trauma

Usually blunt trauma, often associated with other injuries. The liver and spleen are most commonly affected. Gut trauma may result in rupture of the viscus, e.g. duodenum or ileum. Injury to the kidney is common. Pelvic fractures are associated with urinary tract damage. Symptoms may be slow to evolve; major haemorrhage can occur. Gastric dilation is common in major trauma. Useful investigations include:

- abdominal X-ray
- computed tomography
- peritoneal lavage.

Thermal injury

Burns

Scalds and burns are some of the commonest severe injuries in children. These frequently occur at home following spillage of hot fluids, or house fires. Many burn injuries are considered preventable. Electrical burns, in particular, can cause more damage than is initially apparent.

Burn damage is estimated according to the area affected and the depth of the burns, e.g., first, second or third degree burns. Charts are available to help estimate body surface area (BSA) affected. The contribution of the head to surface area is greater in the young than the adult: 18% in the baby versus 9% in the adult.

A severe burn is defined as > 15% BSA affected, or involving the face or perineum.

Early management
Assessment:

- Apply basic ABC of resuscitation.
- Smoke inhalation or airway burns. If this has occurred, early intubation is advisable as swelling rapidly increases after injury and intubation becomes increasingly difficult. Tracheostomy may be necessary, either urgently to manage the airway, or for long-term ventilation.
- Carbon monoxide (CO) inhalation is suggested by decreasing conscious level, 'cherry red' skin and mucous membranes, high carboxyhaemoglobin levels (> 5%) and tissue hypoxia (preferential binding of CO to haemoglobin to form carboxyhaemoglobin). If carboxyhaemoglobin level is > 20%, coma is usually present. Ventilation with 100% O_2 required. Occasionally hyperbaric oxygen therapy is used.
- Fluids are given on the basis of clinical assessment guided by fluid requirement protocols. These protocols vary but all advocate use of large volumes of colloid, blood and blood products, to avoid hypovolaemia, anaemia and coagulopathy with ongoing losses. Volumes are adjusted to the percentage of the body surface area affected by the burn. For example, the Parkland formula recommends IV fluids (Ringer's lactate, or a mixture of crystalloid and colloid) 3–4 ml/kg/day/% body surface area burned for the first 24 h. Half is given over the first 8 h and the rest over the following 16 h. In addition, routine maintenance fluids are required. Fluid requirements are often underestimated and additional fluids needed.
- Protein losses are severe and continuous.
- Vascular access may be difficult; intraosseous needle may be required.
- Direct tissue damage may result in massive haemolysis or rhabdomyolysis causing renal damage.
- Catheterization and careful fluid balance is essential. Aim for urine output of 1–2 ml/kg/h.
- Early surgical escharotomy.
- Transfer to a specialist burns centre may be necessary.

Emergency procedures include debridement of wounds, fasciotomy, and skin grafting. Specific anaesthetic considerations include:

- Suxamethonium is contraindicated due to risk of hyperkalaemia.
- Monitoring can be difficult due to limited access; central venous pressure may be essential to guide fluid management of extensive burns. Third space losses and blood loss can be great.

- Analgesic requirements are high.
- Acute gastric dilation; a nasogastric tube is required.
- Heat losses are great. Humidification, increased ambient temperature and warming IV fluids are useful strategies.
- Sterility must be maintained to prevent infection. Antibiotics and tetanus immunization will be required.

Later management
Debridement of wounds and changing burns dressings usually require general anaesthesia in the child. Later, skin grafting and reconstructive surgery may be necessary.

Important anaesthetic issues include
- Blood loss may be substantial; cross-match required.
- Difficulties with airway management, vascular access, positioning due to scarred tissues and contractures.
- Suxamethonium contraindicated for at least 3 months post-injury.
- Psychological damage, phobic symptoms.
- Pain management.
- Infection, sepsis.

Hypothermia
Classically, this is better tolerated physiologically in the child than the adult, but infants and babies are very vulnerable to cold injury as their protective systems are poorly developed. Most injuries result from cold water immersion or exposure in cold climates. Effects of hypothermia include:

- confusion, lethargy, decreased tendon reflexes
- peripheral vasoconstriction
- decreased renal function
- an initial tachycardia followed by bradycardia with prolonged Q-T, J waves, or atrial dysrhythmia; occasionally ventricular tachycardia
- increased blood viscosity, thrombocytopenia, DIC.

Elective hypothermia is used in cardiac surgery in the repair of some complex lesions. A temperature of 16°C allows circulatory arrest for approximately 60 min during surgery. However, complications increase in severity and incidence with increasing duration of hypothermia.

Elective hypothermia is better tolerated in neonates than in older children. Regardless of the aetiology, rewarming should be slow and even to prevent reperfusion injury.

Methods for rewarming include:

- environmental warming
- warming fluids and inspired gases
- peritoneal dialysis
- use of cardiac bypass.

Transport of the paediatric patient

As paediatric services are being concentrated in designated centres, the need to transfer patients increases. This often involves transfer to specialist units, e.g. burns unit or paediatric intensive care unit.

Transfer of sick children to paediatric intensive care areas is usually done by specialized multidisciplinary transport teams. This provides mobile intensive care support during transfer.

Many forms of transport may be used and distances covered may be considerable. Before transfer, regardless of the reason for transfer, the child should have:

- a secure airway
- stable vital signs
- suitable monitoring in place
- adequate venous access
- received fluid resuscitation
- any wounds covered or stabilized
- notes/X-rays and laboratory results with the patient.

Neonates and babies are transferred in specialist incubators, which maintain a neutral thermal environment and have a cylinder gas supply for a specialized transport ventilator. Before transfer, all cylinders are checked to ensure sufficient gases are available. In addition, a self-inflating bag should always be taken in case of gas failure. Portable incubators incorporate facilities monitoring that include oxygen saturation, pulse and blood pressure, respiratory rate, FiO_2, ECG, capnography and temperature.

Personnel should be trained in transfer and be familiar with all the equipment. Transfer bags must be designed to ensure a sufficient range of equipment sizes is available, from infancy to teenagers.

Contents of a transfer pack include:

- equipment for airway management
- suction equipment

- IV supplies, cannulae (including intraosseous needles) and fluids
- monitoring equipment
- stethoscope
- necessary drugs for sedation, analgesia, inotropic support and muscle relaxation.

16

Sedation

Many procedures, which are done in the awake adult, require general anaesthesia in a child particularly if they involve the child remaining still for long periods or if they are painful. However, there is increasing interest in the use of sedative regimens in paediatrics. This is because it is less invasive than general anaesthesia and cheaper.

Definition

Sedation is the use of drugs to produce a state of depression of the central nervous system to allow treatment to be undertaken. During treatment, verbal contact with the patient must be maintained.

Using this definition, any loss of consciousness associated with the technique is defined as general anaesthesia. During sedation, the patient is expected to maintain an airway and protective reflexes. The concept of 'deep sedation' has been suggested, but the definition of this state is not clear. It may be particularly difficult in the young child to determine the level of sedation and there is a danger that anaesthesia may result.

Recent guidelines from the Department of Health on general anaesthesia and dentistry recommended more use of conscious sedation and local anaesthesia, reserving the use of general anaesthesia for when absolutely necessary.

If patients are carefully selected, and the procedures are appropriate, sedation can be very successful (see Box 16.1). All sedation services should provide:

- Trained staff and dedicated assistants. These may include medical and dental staff, nurses and operating department personnel, who must all be appropriately trained in the theoretical and clinical aspects of sedation and be clear about their role.
- The person doing the procedure is defined as the 'operator' and a separate trained person administers sedation and cares for the child during the procedure, the 'sedationist'.

- Systems for the organization of care of patients including:
  - preoperative assessment, pre- and postoperative information
  - fasting protocols
  - a process for obtaining informed consent.
- Suitable, well-maintained equipment and monitoring should be available. Minimum monitoring includes conscious level, pain, respiratory rate and pattern, pulse rate and colour. If IV sedation is used, pulse oximetry is standard and for many procedures blood pressure, capnography, electrocardiogram and temperature are increasingly used routinely.
- Resuscitation facilities.
- Training in basic life support, and ideally in advanced life support.
- Regular practice in resuscitation skills.
- Staff trained to assist in the management of medical emergencies.
- Data records and audit of practice.

Box 16.1   Procedures that may be undertaken with sedation

Dental extractions, conservations	Radiology: CT scans, MRI, angiography
Insertion of vascular catheters	
Cardiac catheterization	Lumbar puncture, bone marrow aspirates, oesophagogastroscopy
Minor suturing, removal of sutures	
Dressings, e.g. for burns	Removal/change of plasters
	Joint injections
	Muscle biopsy
	Transcutaneous biopsy, e.g. renal, hepatic

Contraindications to sedation

- Patient refusal/parent refusal.
- Small babies having non-painful procedures, e.g. computed tomography, can usually be fed and kept warm so that they sleep during the procedure. They should not be sedated.
- Expremature babies < 56 weeks' post conceptional age, due to a risk of respiratory depression and excess sedation.
- Severe behavioural disorders.
- Known airway problems, e.g. obstructive sleep apnoea, craniofacial abnormalities.

- Significant respiratory disease requiring oxygen therapy.
- Significant cardiac instability.
- Marked renal or hepatic disease which would prevent predictable clearance of sedative drugs.
- Significant risk of gastro-oesophageal reflux.
- Raised intracranial pressure.
- Severe or poorly controlled epilepsy.
- Allergy or specific contraindication to sedative drugs or gases (e.g. nitrous oxide is avoided if a pneumothorax is present).
- Prolonged or painful procedure.

Drugs used for sedation

Many institutions have carefully designed drug regimens which are successful. Effective sedation should allow the procedure to be undertaken whilst the child is drowsy, pain free, with minimal fear or anxiety. The use of local anaesthesia and simple analgesics is important, and distraction therapy is also very useful. Parents are frequently able to be present, which is helpful in maintaining the confidence of the child.

Most sedative drugs, given in sufficient amounts, risk producing unconsciousness in the child. This may result in hypoxia, hypercapnia and potential aspiration. If non-anaesthetists are using sedation techniques, then the margin of safety must be large.

Non-anaesthetic personnel providing sedation include physicians (particularly radiologists, gastroenterologists and cardiologists), specialist nurses and dentists, all of whom must be fully trained to provide a safe and effective service.

The organization of sedation for children within hospital is evolving rapidly. Some paediatric centres train sedationists who are usually specialist nurses (nurse-lead sedation). However, the responsibility for training and development should ideally lie with the anaesthetic department with a named consultant overseeing the service.

Patients should be prepared as though they were having a general anaesthetic.

They should:

- be informed of the process and have given consent
- be fasted
- have their general health reviewed, identifying any potential risk factors such as allergies or medical conditions.

Oral drugs

Doses of oral drugs can be difficult to judge and combinations of drugs, whilst increasing the likelihood of effective sedation, also increase the potential for side effects (see Box 16.2). This is particularly true in small babies and in children with abnormal renal, hepatic or neurological function when the action of drugs may be unpredictable (see Box 16.3 and 16.4).

Recovery and reversal

Recovery from sedation should be rapid. Full recovery facilities must be available. Most drug regimens are short acting. However, reversal of benzodiazepines may be necessary. Flumazenil 1–2 μg/kg IV is used. Occasionally, naloxone is required to antagonize persistent opioid effect. Naloxone 4 μg/kg IV is given.

Box 16.2   Oral sedation agents

Drug	Sedation dose, orally (mg/kg)	Details
Chloral hydrate	100	Active metabolite = trichlorethanol
		Can be given rectally
		Occasional disinhibition
Triclofos	50–75 max 1 g	Active metabolite = trichlorethanol
Trimeprazine	2	Higher doses may cause 'grey baby syndrome'
Midazolam	0.5–1.0	Commonly used
		Dose related side effects (ataxia, double vision, sedation)
		Can also be given nasally, rectally dose may vary
Diazepam	200–500 mcg/kg	Can be given rectally
Ketamine	5–10	Can be given also nasally, rectally
		Hallucinations may occur
		nausea and vomiting (N&V) common
		Apnoea may occur

Note: in larger children doses should not exceed normal adult doses.

Box 16.3   Intravenous sedation agents

Drug	Sedation dose (mg/kg)	Details
Midazolam	0.05–0.2	Apnoea may occur Amnesia Disinhibited behaviour may occur
Diazepam	0.1–0.5	Diazemuls = lipid formulation Long half life, risk of delayed recovery
Fentanyl diazepam,	0.5 mcg/kg	Used with propofol, midazolam or ketamine Can be used transorally Apnoea, N&V may occur Potentiates effect of other sedatives
Ketamine	0.5–1.0	Can be given IM, orally, IV Frequently used with benzodiazepines
Propofol	Undergoing evaluation	Risk of apnoea Risk of inducing anaesthesia

Box 16.4   Inhalational sedation agents

Agent	Dose	Details
Nitrous oxide	50% N_2O in O_2 (entonox)	Provides analgesia
	70% in O_2	Requires patient cooperation Nausea common Dysphoria
Sevoflurane	1% in air	Undergoing evaluation

Further reading

Scottish Intercollegiate Guidelines Network. Safe sedation of children undergoing diagnostic and therapeutic procedures. Online. Available: www.sign.au.uk

A conscious decision. A review of the use of general anaesthesia and conscious sedation in primary dental care. Department of Health Publications. Online. Available:www.doh.gov.uk/dental/conscious.htm

17

Anaesthesia for procedures outside the operating theatre

There has been rapid growth in the numbers of paediatric patients requiring general anaesthesia or sedation outside the operating room (Box 17.1). Sedation can be used for some of these procedures but general anaesthesia is still necessary for many.

Box 17.1 Procedures occurring outside the operating theatre

Diagnostic and interventional imaging procedures that may require general anaesthesia	• MRI • CT scanning, CT guided biopsies • Neuroradiology • Angiography, e.g. cardiac and neurosurgery • Echocardiography • Interventional radiology
Medical procedures	• Lumbar puncture • Intrathecal injections • Bone marrow aspiration • Insertion of percutaneous long-term venous access (PICC line) • Upper or lower gastrointestinal endoscopy • Renal and liver biopsies • Joint injections
Therapeutic interventions	• Radiation therapy

General anaesthesia requires the same standards of preoperative assessment, equipment, monitoring, recovery and skilled assistance regardless of location. As these procedures occur in remote sites, it is essential that an experienced anaesthetist is present.

Magnetic resonance imaging (MRI)

MRI scans are extensively used in paediatrics, particularly for the investigation of neurological disease, metabolic problems, tumours, epilepsy, cardiac disease and trauma. Several aspects of MRI scanning make it difficult to scan small or uncooperative children without sedation or anaesthesia:

- Scanner environment: the area into which the patient is placed to obtain the scans is a long, narrow tube which is frightening for small children.
- Noise: while the scanner is acquiring images it is very noisy (> 90 db).
- Time: newer scanners still take 15–20 min to obtain a routine brain scan. More complex sequences may take longer.
- Immobility: it is important that during acquisition sequences the patient is completely still.

Recently, 'open' scanners have been developed which do not have a confining tunnel. It is possible for older, cooperative children to go into such a scanner without anaesthesia or sedation. However, most children will require either sedation or general anaesthesia, although very young infants < 4 weeks can be 'fed and wrapped' as they tend to go to fall asleep and can then be scanned.

Department design, equipment and monitoring

Department design

The design of MRI units is crucial to the successful running of anaesthetic and sedation services.

Ideal design characteristics include the provision of an anaesthetic room, an adjacent recovery room and a sedation area. Decisions should also be made about whether day cases will be admitted to the unit itself or to another day care area. Another important design consideration is where the anaesthetist is expected to be while the child is in the scanner: in the scanning room or outside.

Most anaesthetists prefer to be outside as it is very noisy in the scanner and it is prudent to avoid overexposure to the magnetic field. If the anaesthetic room is designed to have a door and window into the scanner the anaesthetist can remain in the anaesthetic room with a good view of the patient, the monitoring and the anaesthetic machine.

Monitoring and equipment

Specially designed anaesthetic monitors are required for use in the MRI scanner, as all cables and connectors must be non-ferrous.

- The pulse oximeter is usually fibreoptic and the electrocardiogram cables are carbon fibre.

- The blood pressure cuffs and tubing have non-ferrous connectors. Problems may arise in very small infants where the length of tubing means that the compressible volume in the tubes is too large to transmit the small pulse pressure.
- Capnography is useful but there is a short delay in response because of the long tubing.
- There is equipment available to monitor invasive pressures during scanning but transducers from the paediatric intensive care unit (PICU) are usually ferrous and need to be replaced.

If the child becomes unstable or arrests while in the scanner, there are two choices. One is to deal with the patient in the scanner, the second is to transfer the child to the anaesthetic room for further management. The authors prefer to deal with these situations outside the scanner. This has the advantage that all equipment required during acute management does not need to be non-ferrous.

Anaesthetic considerations
General anaesthesia
- General anaesthesia and sedation lists should be run separately, and not mixed.
- Patients with a wide range of serious medical problems present for MRI. Careful preoperative assessment is essential.
- The majority of patients will be admitted as day cases, although some will already be in hospital and some may be ventilated in PICU.
- Patients must have a 'metal check' before entering the scanner.
- Sedative premedication is generally not required.
- Local anaesthetic cream is useful if IV induction is planned.
- Inhalational or IV induction is suitable. Propofol is used for IV induction and some anaesthetists also use it for maintenance.
- Most children breathe spontaneously using an LMA. Small infants (< 3 kg) should probably be intubated and ventilated.
- It may be necessary to give IV MRI contrast medium. The incidence of allergic reactions to this contrast is much lower that to X-ray contrast.
- Postanaesthesia delirium is common if volatile anaesthetics are used as the sole anaesthetic agent.

Computed tomography (CT) scanning
There are generally fewer requirements for anaesthesia in the CT scanner compared with the MRI scanner.

More children are able to undergo a CT scan without sedation or anaesthesia because:

- A CT scan is quick. Even complex investigations only take a few minutes and immobility is required for only short periods.
- CT scanners are quiet.
- The area where the child is placed is more like a doughnut than a tunnel and is much less frightening.

Anaesthetic considerations
- Spontaneously breathing techniques with LMA are usually adequate.
- IV contrast may be required. Reactions are rare but all appropriate drugs and equipment including a defibrillator must be readily available.
- The anaesthetic machine and monitors are in the scanning area and the anaesthetist usually remains in the scanner.

Angiography
Cerebral, renal and cardiac angiography in children usually require general anaesthesia. The sites at which angiography take place are usually remote from the main operating theatres, so help in an emergency may be delayed. It is important that these areas are fully equipped and that the anaesthetists are experienced.

Cerebral angiography
Cerebral angiography may be diagnostic or therapeutic. In the latter case, embolization of arteriovenous malformations is achieved with a coil or glue.

Careful preoperative assessment is required. Particular attention should be paid to:

- Conscious level of the child.
- Features of raised intracranial pressure.
- If an intracranial arteriovenous shunt is present the child may have a bruit and high-output cardiac failure.
- In stroke, a procoagulant abnormality such as protein C deficiency may be present. Advice from haematologists should be sought.
- Potential causes of embolization, such as congenital heart disease or endocarditis, should be considered.

Anaesthetic considerations
- Sedative premedication is avoided.

- General anaesthesia with tracheal intubation and controlled ventilation is used.
- Access to the patient is limited. Long extensions for IV cannulae and long ventilator tubing are required.
- Monitoring of core temperature is necessary and active heating with warm air blankets or other means is used to maintain body temperature.
- Vascular access, arterial and venous, is usually achieved via the femoral vessels. Local anaesthesia is useful for insertion of these cannulae. Opiates are usually unnecessary.
- Intravenous contrast produces an osmotic diuresis and postoperative IV fluids are necessary.

After the procedure:

- Adequate recovery facilities should be available.
- Bleeding from the femoral puncture sites is a risk, particularly in small babies in whom large blood volumes can be lost rapidly.

Intravenous contrast media

Intravenous contrast media is iodine based and should not be used in those with an allergy to iodine. Both ionic and non-ionic forms are made but the non-ionic form is preferred in children. If ionic dyes are used then a 30% or 60% solution should be selected. Non-allergic reactions to the dye can occur with flushing, tachycardia or nausea, probably a result of the hyperosmolar nature of the dyes. True allergic reactions may also occur even without prior exposure, or a history of iodine allergy. The high osmolarity of the dyes (ionic > non-ionic) and the high sodium content of the ionic compound result in an osmotic diuresis that causes a reduction in the intravascular volume. Intravenous fluids should be given during the procedure to maintain the intravascular volume of the child and should also be given postoperatively until drinking is restored. The recommended maximum dose of ionic dyes is 5 ml/kg and of non-ionic dyes 4 ml/kg.

Radiotherapy

Most children will require general anaesthesia to undergo radiotherapy.

- Radiotherapy usually takes place at least once but perhaps twice a day for several consecutive days.

It is important that the confidence of the child is maintained throughout the treatment.

- The choice of anaesthetic depends on the patient and on the area treated. General anaesthesia with an LMA and spontaneous breathing is used, as is sedation with a propofol infusion. Many patients have a Hickman line, which makes IV administration easy. Ketamine is used infrequently because of the risk of hallucinations and slower recovery times.
- If the head is the target of the therapy, the child is placed in a specially made mask which is held in a frame. This makes access to the airway difficult.
- Very high doses of radiation are used and it is not possible for medical personnel to remain in the treatment room. Closed circuit television is required to see the patient.

Medical procedures

An increasing number of medical procedures are required in children, particularly in association with oncology. The use of an operating room is unnecessary. The development of a specially designed procedure area, which may be attached to an oncology ward, is safe and efficient for these minor procedures.

An admission area, procedure room with anaesthetic machine and monitors, well-trained staff and a recovery ward, and an area to wait before discharge are essential.

Accidental intrathecal injection of toxic drugs continues to occur in adults and children. Clear protocols must be in place to reduce the possibility of inadvertent intrathecal injection.

Anaesthetic considerations

- Most patients are day cases.
- Many patients come for repeated procedures.
- Patients undergoing chemotherapy need a full blood count to determine white cell and platelet numbers before lumber puncture or bone marrow.
- Many patients have long-term, tunnelled venous catheters (Hickman line, PICC line or Portacath), which can be used for induction and/or maintenance of anaesthesia.
- These procedures are very rapid and postoperative pain is not usually a problem. It is frequently sufficient to use a bolus dose of propofol in combination with a short-acting opioid such as remifentanil or

alfentanil with the child breathing oxygen alone. This ensures that the patient is unconscious and pain free during the procedure but recovers very quickly.

- Some patients without IV access may prefer inhalational induction.
- Ketamine is now used less frequently because of the risk of hallucinations. Children who come for repeated procedures dislike ketamine.

Use of tunnelled central venous catheters

- Great care is necessary
  - aseptic technique must be used
  - adequate flush after use; 20 ml saline 0.9%.
- Beware heparin. Some units use heparin (1000 units per ml) in the catheter to prevent clotting, in which case the catheter must be aspirated before use. At the end of the procedure, the precise volume of heparin should be replaced.

18

Resuscitation

Guidelines for the resuscitation of infants and children have been issued by the European Resuscitation Council. These have taken into account the evidence-based information from the International Liaison Committee on Resuscitation (ILCOR).

Aetiology

The causes of cardiorespiratory arrest in the young are different from adult practice. Whereas ventricular fibrillation or cardiac dysrhythmias are the commonest cause of arrest in adults, these are rare in children. Children tend to have primarily a respiratory cause for arrest resulting in increasing hypoxia and eventually profound acidosis, bradycardia and cardiac arrest (see Box 18.1). Therefore, children have a longer period of gradual decline when treatment has a good chance of averting arrest. Unfortunately, as the period of deterioration may be long, the child may become severely damaged physiologically, and although resuscitation may be achieved the likelihood of permanent damage, particularly neurological, is increased.

Causes of arrest

The cause of paediatric arrests differs between neonates and babies/children and also between those that occur in hospital and in the community. The eventual outcome is also different.

Main causes of arrest in childhood
Respiratory:

- aspiration of foreign body
- croup/epiglottitis
- sudden infant death syndrome (SIDS)
- asthma.

Accidents:

- drowning
- road traffic accidents (RTAs)
- head trauma
- non-accidental injury
- poisoning.

Other:

- cardiac arrhythmias, e.g. in children with cardiac disease
- sepsis
- meningitis
- seizures
- electrolyte disorder, metabolic disease.

Trauma causes half the deaths in 1–14 year age group:

- 50% RTA
- 25% falls
- 15% burns.

Box 18.1   Signs and symptoms indicating potential cardiorespiratory arrest in the paediatric patient

Respiratory	Cardiovascular	CNS	Other
• Apnoea	• Arrhythmias particularly bradycardia	• Disorientation	• Cyanosis
• Grunting		• Lethargy	• Mottling
• Tachypnoea		• Irritability	• Sweating
• Retraction of respiratory muscles	• Decreased blood pressure		• Evidence of dehydration
• Nasal flaring	• Sluggish capillary refill		

Factors to consider when treating the critically ill child include:

- altered conscious level – record Glasgow Coma Score
- haemodynamic instability

- altered drug metabolism in the shocked patient
- delayed stomach emptying.

Outcome

Overall survival is 14% (survival for out-of-hospital arrest is 7% and 22% for in-hospital arrest).

Success depends on the cause of the arrest and the location, (pre-hospital, hospital, intensive care units). The quality of outcome also varies.

Causes of arrest in babies < 1 month old

- congenital abnormalities
- SIDS
- trauma.

Resuscitation of the newborn

Apgar scoring is the initial assessment used following delivery (see Box 18.2). It is checked at 1, 5 and 10 min. Low apgars < 6 at 1 min indicate asphyxia and likely acidosis, except in very low birth weight babies in whom low scores are not necessarily associated with asphyxia. Apgars < 3 indicate severe asphyxia. These babies need active resuscitation.

Box 18.2   Apgar score assessment

Sign	Scores		
	0	1	2
Heart rate	None	< 100 bpm	< 100 bpm
Respiratory effort	None	Slow/irregular	Good
Muscle tone	Limp	Some flexion	Active
Reflex irritability	No response	Grimace	Cough or sneeze
Colour	Pale/blue	Body pink, limbs blue	pink

Management includes:

- Dry and warm the baby.
- Clear the airway, give oxygen.
- Use a bag, mask and airway to assist ventilation.
- Chest compressions if the heart rate is less than 100. This is best assessed by feeling the umbilical or axillary artery or for cardiac pulsations directly on the chest.

- Further management includes establishing IV access, administration of adrenaline (epinephrine), volume (0.9% sodium chloride), glucose, if hypoglycaemia is present, and sodium bicarbonate to treat acidosis.

Paediatric life support
Basic life support (BLS)
shout for help
evaluate ABC
check for response.

AIRWAY
- Head tilt/chin lift.
- Remove visible foreign matter.

BREATHING
- Start mouth to mouth respiration if no respiratory effort in 10 sec (mouth to nose in infants).
- Give oxygen if possible.

CIRCULATION
- Check the carotid or brachial artery.
- Start chest compressions early if heart rate < 60, or there are signs of poor perfusion.

Figures 18.1 and 18.2 present algorithms for paediatric basic and advanced life support.

Equipment required for resuscitation
- suction.
- guedel airways and face masks of various sizes and types.
- self-inflating bags, e.g. AMBU; these are made in three sizes:
  - neonatal   240 ml
  - child   500 ml
  - adult   1600 ml.

If necessary, the larger bags can be used on small patients as long as care is taken to watch the movement of the chest with each ventilation, to ensure that it is not excessive.

- Laryngoscopes.
- LMAs™.
- Selection of tracheal tubes, (in an emergency chose a tracheal tube approximately the external diameter of the child's fifth finger).
- Bougie/stylet
- Venous catheters, IV fluids.
- Intraosseous needle.
- Other syringes, wipes, nasogastric tubes.
- Monitoring: ECG, SPO_2, NIBP, $ETCO_2$, temperature.
- Emergency tracheastomy set.
- Although cooling confers cerebral protection, unfortunately small children and babies lose heat excessively. Warmed covers, overhead heaters, warming IV fluids and maintaining high ambient temperature are important.
- Hypothermia is tolerated better in children that adults. Full recovery has been reported after circulatory arrest in cold environments.
- Broselow tape which aids correct choice of drug doses by correlating a guessed weight from the measured length of the child.
- Algorithms for resuscitation, e.g. The European Resuscitation Council, The Oakley Chart.

Further reading

Richmond CE, Bingham RM. Paediatric cardiopulmonary resuscitation. *Paediatric Anaesthesia* 1995; 5:11–27.

Phillips B, Ziderman D et al. European resuscitation council guidelines 2000 for paediatric basic life support. *Resuscitation* 2000;48:223–229.

Phillips B, Ziderman D et al. European resuscitation council guidelines 2000 for paediatric advanced life support. *Resuscitation* 2000;48:231–234.

American Heart Association in Collaboration with the International Liaison Committee on Resuscitation (ILCOR) Guidelines 2000 for Cardiorespiratory Resuscitation and Emergency Cardiovascular Care-An International Consensus on Science. (a) *Resuscitation* 2000;46:301–99, (b) *Circulation* 2000;102:11–384.

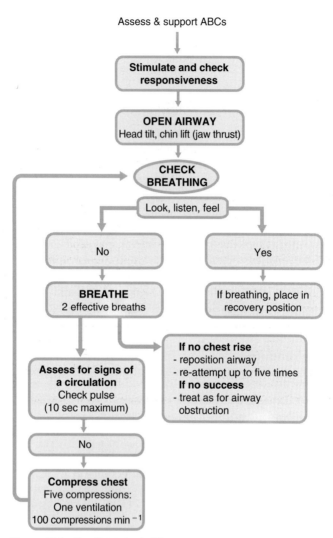

Figure 18.1   Paediatric basic life support.

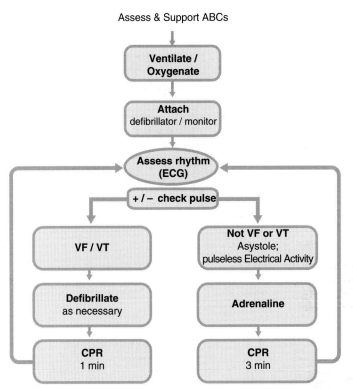

Figure 18.2 Paediatric advanced life support – CPR, Cardiopulmonary resuscitation.

Box 18.3 During advanced cardiopulmonary resuscitation

- **Check**
  - Tracheal tube placement
  - Vascular access
  - ECG placement

- **Defibrillate**
  - Initially 2 J/kg, 2 J/kg, 4 J/kg, subsequently 4 J/kg × 3

- **Give adrenaline (epinephrine) every 3 min**
  - **IV/IO** 0.01 mg/kg (1:10,000; 0.1 ml/kg)
  - **Tracheal** 0.1 mg/kg (1:1000; 0.1 ml/kg)

- **Consider using antiarrythmic drugs** eg.
  - **Amiodarone** 5 mg/kg bolus IV/IO **OR**
  - **Lignocaine** 1 mg/kg bolus IV/IO/PT **OR**
  - **Magnesium** 25–50 mg/kg IV/IO for or torsades de pointes hypomagnesemia (max: 2g)

- **Consider giving sodium bicarbonate 8.4%**
  - 1 ml/kg

- **Correct potentially reversible causes**
  - Hypoxaemia
  - Hypovolaemia
  - Hypothermia
  - Hyper +/– hypokalemia and metabolic disorders
  - Tamponade
  - Tension pneumothorax
  - Thromboembolism
  - Toxins/poisons/drugs

19

Web pages

The following are useful web addresses related to paediatric anaesthesia.

General
The Association of Anaesthetists of Great Britain and Ireland: http:/www.aagbi.org

Paediatric information
General information: http://pedsanesthesia.stanford.edu/

Syndromes
Online Mendelian Inheritance in Man: http://www.ncbi.nlm.nih.gov/ Omim/
Paediatric cardiology site: http://www.Kumc.edu/kumcpeds/
Neonatal site: http://www.neonatology.org/index.html
Information on the paediatric pain management: http://www.ich.ucl.ac. uk/cpap/

Organizations
Society of Pediatric Anaesthesia: http://www.pedsanesthesia.org
Association of Paediatric Anaesthetists of Great Britain and Ireland: http://www.apagbi.org.uk
European Resuscitation Council: http://www.erc.edu
Resuscitation Council (UK): http://www.resus.org.uk
Scottish Intercollegiate Guidelines Network (sedation): http://www.sign.ac.uk

Index